HERBAL MEDIC NEUROPSYCHIATRIC DISEASES

Current Developments and Research

HERBAL MEDICINES FOR NEUROPSYCHIATRIC DISEASES

Current Developments and Research

Edited by

Shigenobu Kanba, M.D., Ph.D.
Department of Neuropsychiatry, Yamanashi Medical University

and

Elliott Richelson, M.D., Ph.D.
Department of Research, Mayo Clinic Jacksonville

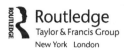

Routledge
Taylor & Francis Group
New York London

First published by BRUNNER / MAZEL PUBLISHERS Philadelphia & London

This edition published 2012 by Routledge

Routledge
Taylor & Francis Group
711 Third Avenue
New York, NY 10017

Routledge
Taylor & Francis Group
27 Church Road
Hove East Sussex BN3 2FA

HERBAL MEDICINES FOR NEUROPSYCHIATRIC DISEASES : Current Developments and Research

A CIP catalog record for this book is available from the British Library.

Library of Congress Cataloging-in-Publication Data

Herbal medicines for neuropsychiatric diseases : current developments and research/edited by Shigenobu
    Kanba and Elliott Richelson.
        p.   cm.
    Includes bibliographical references and indexes.
    ISBN 0-87630-804-3
        1. Herbs-Therapeutic use. 2. Neuropsychopharmacology. 3. Nervous system—Diseases—
Chemotherapy. 4. Mental illness—Chemotherapy. 1. Kanba, Shigenobu. II. Richelson, Elliott.
        [DNLM : 1. Mental Disorders—drug therapy. 2. Nervous System Diseases—drug therapy. 3. Plant
Extracts—therapeutic use. 4. Plant Extracts—pharmacology. 5. Medicine, Herbal. WM403H534 1998]
RC350.H47H47   1998
616.8'0461—dc21
DNLM/DLC
for Library of Congress
                                                                                                              98-45054
0-87630-804-3   CIP

CONTENTS

CONTRIBUTORS

Jerry Cott, Ph.D.
Division of Clinical and Treatment Research
National Institute of Mental Health
Rockville, MD 20857
U.S.A

B.N. Dhawan, M.D., F.N.A.
ICMR Center for Advanced Pharmacological
Research on Traditional Remedies
Central Drug Research Institute
PB No. 173
Lucknow 226001
India

Shigenobu Kanba, M.D.
Department of Neuropsychiatry
Yamanashi Medical University,
Yamanashi, 409-3821
Japan

Masao Kishikawa, M.D., Ph.D.
Department of Pathology, Scientific Data
Center for the Atomic Bomb Disaster
Nagasaki University School of Medicine
Nagasaki 852-8102
Japan

A.P. Kozikowski, Ph.D.
Georgetown University
Washington, D.C.
U.S.A.

M. McKinney, Ph.D.
Department of Pharmacology
Mayo Clinic Jacksonville
Jacksonville, FL 32224
U.S.A.

Renuka Misra, Ph.D.
National Institute on Aging
National Institute of Health
Baltimore, MD 21224
U.S.A.

Otto Sticher, Ph.D.
Department of Pharmacy
Federal Institute of Technology (ETH) Zurich
CH-8057,
Zurich
Switzerland

Kiminobu Sugaya, Ph.D.
Department of Pharmacology
Mayo Clinic Jacksonville
Jacksonville, FL 32224
U.S.A.

X.C. Tang
State Key Laboratory of Drug Research
Shanghai
Institute of Materia Medica
Chinese Academy of Sciences
Shanghai 200031
China

Kazuo Yamada, M.D., Takaaki Murata, M.D. Hiroko Mizushima, M.D.
Masahiro Asai, M.D.
Department of Herbal Medicine
Keio University School of Medicine
Tokyo 160-0016
Japan

Zuxin Wang, M.D. Guiying Ren Ph.D., Youwen Zhao, M.D. Yaqin Weng, M.D. Mingchen Ding, M.D. Xinqing Zhang, M.D. Chen Meng, M.D. Peijie Yang, M.D. Zhongxuan Wu, M.D. Jianping Wang, M.D. Baozhu Li, M.D. Yunru Zhang, M.D. Ruicheng Hau, M.D. Jianan Wei, M.D. Shuzhen Huang, M.D. Shuhua Fei, M.D. Baorong Fan, M.D. Shulan Wang, M.D. Xiangping Ma, M.D. Qian Xia, M.D.
Institute of Mental Health
Beijing Medical University
Beijing 100083 PRC

Introduction: Integrating the Old and the New

The impetus for this book was a symposium on the development of new neuropsychiatric drugs from traditional herbal medicines, held at the 19th Collegium Internationale Neuro-psychopharmacologicum (CINP) Congress on July 1, 1994, in Washington, D.C. The symposium, cochaired by the author and Dr. Shigenobu Kanba of the Yamanashi Medical University in Yamanashi, brought together a group of distinguished scientists from around the world to discuss the role that ages-old medicinals can play in modern-day therapy.

For the participants, in general, the subject did not represent a revolution (although perhaps, for a few, an evolution) in their scientific thinking. Most came from countries where herbal medicines not only have been used for centuries, but are still being utilized by mainstream practitioners as valid forms of therapy. An important exception, of course, is the United States, which requires that for a drug to be prescribed for human use, its chemistry and pharmacology must be precisely defined, and it must meet governmental standards for safety and efficacy—which could pose an obstacle to the speedy approval of drugs based on what some might label folkloric remedies.

Nevertheless, many U.S. scientists strongly support the concept that herbal medicines offer enormous possibilities for the discovery of new drugs, particularly in light of the inadequacy of our current pharmacology to treat neuropsychiatric disorders.

The relevance of this endorsement by Western professionals is reflected in our opening chapter, which was written by researchers from the U.S. National Institutes of Health. In "Medicinal Plants: A Potential Source of New Psychotherapeutic Drugs," they describe programs already under way in the United States to investigate how these traditional medicines might provide the basis for new, more effective psychopharmacology. In contrast, the next three chapters go back to the ancient cultures of Japan, China, and India, respectively, to present the perspective—past, present, and future—on herbal medicines in those countries. Other chapters are narrower in focus: the complex chemistry of ginkgo, a Chinese shade tree with edible berries that hold promise as an adjunct therapy for the elderly; the in vitro pharmacology of himbacine; a muscarinic antagonist, and huperzine A, a potent and selective acetylcholinesterase inhibitor, both of which are active ingredients of natural products; and the results of controlled clinical trial with huperzine A from China, where the compound was first discovered. To round out the picture, the final two chapters are devoted to reports of studies in which behavioral and biochemical effects of various herbal preparations were tested on senescence-acclerated mice.

For clinical and basic scientists alike, this book will provide an overview of the status of traditional herbal medicines as they relate to the treatment of neuropsychiatric diseases today. It will also serve as a source for some detailed information on specific natural products and their constituents, as well as a reference point at which to begin a more in-depth exploration of this fascinating field.

Elliott Richelson, M.D.

HERBAL MEDICINES FOR NEUROPSYCHIATRIC DISEASES

Current Developments and Research

1

Use of Herbal Medicine for Treating Psychiatric Disorders in Japan

Shigenobu Kanba, Kazuo Yamada, Hiroko Mizushima, Takaaki Murata, and Masahiro Asai

Although Western pharmacotherapy is now the major medical modality in Japan, traditional remedies are still being offered. Research into traditional treatments continues, and a number of studies have described the basic pharmacology and clinical efficacy of Oriental herbal medicine (Kampo medicine) in Japan.

After being advised of the advantages, as well as the potentially adverse effects, of both herbal and pharmaceutical treatments, patients may choose the approach they prefer. Many patients recognize the limits of the current medical technology and seek more individualized treatments. According to Kampo medicine, health can be preserved by maintaining a prudent lifestyle, eating proper food, and utilizing natural medicines.

INTRODUCTION

As a result of Japan's gradual acceptance of the role of *Kampo* medicine, the Ministry of Health and Welfare now includes such prescriptions in the country's National Health Insurance Plan. About 120 different formulations, which are extracted from combinations of herbs, are available. They also can be prepared in the form of powder.

In a 1993 survey of 2000 physicians by the Japan Medical Association (Fig. 1), 77% reported using *Kampo*, as compared with only 28% in 1979. Common diseases for which *Kampo* is prescribed include hepatitis and liver disease, upper respiratory infections, menopausal syndrome, psychosomatic disorders, allergic rhinitis, constipation, asthma, gastritis, lumbago, and eczema.

About 30 different pharmaceutical companies produce *Kampo* formulations

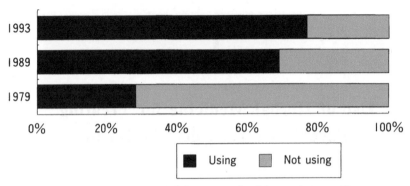

Figure 1. Percentage of Japanese physicians who use *Kampo*. A survey of 2000 physicians by the Japan Medical Association in 1993 revealed that about 77% use *Kampo*, as compared with the 28% reported in 1979.

that are registered by the government. Global sales in 1993 totaled about 1400 billion yen ($14 billion U.S.).

HISTORY OF *KAMPO* MEDICINE

Ancient Chinese medicine traveled to Japan via Korea. It is based on an Oriental philosophy, the yin-yan of taoism. In the year 984, Yasuyori Tamba compiled the *Ishinho*, a vast compendium of Chinese medicine. Later, in the 16th to 18th centuries, three schools of *Kampo* medicine were established.

The Gosei-ha, the first independent school of medicine in Japan, was established when Dosan Manase assembled the various elements of medical theory that had been imported from China since the Sung dynasty. The Koho-ha school arose in reaction to the overly theoretical methodology of the Gosei-ha, and turned back to the ancient medicine of China. Then came the *Setchu-ha*, or compromise, school, which mixed both schools of thought.

Until about 120 years ago, *Kampo* was the official medicine of Japan. Then, strongly influenced by Western culture and civilization, the government decided that Japanese doctors should practice Western medicine and that it should be taught in medical schools. By the end of World War II, the use of *Kampo* had virtually disappeared.

In recent decades, however, *Kampo* medicine has again become popular. Patients, as well as physicians, have reconsidered the value of its holistic and humane aspects. *Kampo* medicine is recognized for its efficacy and safety; moreover, the cost of such treatment may be covered by medical insurance.

BASICS OF *KAMPO* MEDICINE

General Concept

The fundamental philosophy of *Kampo* treatment is the enhancement of the natural healing power. Herbs are believed to affect both the psyche and the soma, and *Kampo* medicine does not differentiate between them. The treatment not only aims at improving or maintaining physical health, but it also takes into account the patient's psychic and mental balance. Futhermore, the human being is regarded as a microcosm reflecting the macrocosm.

The improvement induced by herbal medicine is usually mild and slow, but it can be dramatic. Side effects are rare, and those that do occur are mostly allergic reactions to natural substances. When herbs are combined with interferon to treat chronic hepatitis, there is an increased risk of interstitial pneumonitis.

The specific prescription is traditionally selected by judging the *Sho* of a patient. *Sho* is equivalent to a syndrome, but it comprises psychic and somatic symptoms and signs obtained by a traditional physical examination that focuses on the patient's constitution, general physical condition, pulse, and abdominal signs, and includes an examination of the tongue. A modern diagnosis is also utilized when a prescription is formulated, because most physicians are not trained to determine *Sho* correctly.

Ki-Ketsu-Sui Theory

The *Kampo* concept that is most relevant when treating psychiatric problems is *Ki-Ketsu-Sui* theory. Unhealthy conditions are thought to be caused by the impairment of one, or a combination, of three factors (Terasawa, 1993).

The first factor is *Ki* (*Chi* in Chinese, *Prana* in Aryuveda, *Vis Vitalis* in the traditional European medical system). *Ki* is the basic, all-penetrating, maintaining force or energy, the elemental energy that is the source of all other forms of energy. It is also thought to be the source of nourishment and stimulation for the circulation of body fluids. In addition, *Ki* is responsible for protecting the organism against external and internal noxious forces by circulating as yang-*Ki* in the outer layers of the body.

Disturbances of *Ki* are classified as *Ki* deficiency, *Ki* stasis, or an imbalance of *Ki* distribution. In *Kampo* medicine, depression is considered a *Ki* deficiency or *Ki* stasis. For *Ki* deficiency, *Ninjin-to* or *Keisi-to* is typically indicated. For *Ki* stasis, *Koso-san* and *Hange-koboku-to* are indicated.

Another basic component is *Ketsu*, which is equivalent to blood. According to traditional Chinese medicine, *Ketsu* refers to the red-stained fluid of the organism. A disturbance of *Ketsu* is classified as either a deficiency or a stasis.

Some symptoms caused by a deficiency of *Ketsu* appear in psychiatric disorders. *Shimotsu-to, Kyuki-kyogia-to,* or *Kami-kihi-to* is used to treat this condition.

The third component is *Sui,* body fluid. Statis of *Sui* includes such conditions as palpitations, vertigo, motion sickness, tinnitus, headache, thirst, nausea, emesis, swollen joints in the morning, and a feeling of heaviness in the body.

When a patient, who will often have psychiatric problems, presents with these symptoms, *Ryokei-jutsukan-to* or *Hange-byakujutsu-tenma-to* is indicated.

Ketsuo stasis is often seen in psychiatric patients, especially those who take psychotropic medications. *Teito-to, Tokaku-shoki-to,* and *Kami-shoyo-san* are used to correct these disturbances.

HERBAL MEDICINE FOR PSYCHIATRIC DISORDERS

Animal Studies

A variety of plants are believed to exert central effects. Some plants have been demonstrated to have neuropsychopharmacologic effects.

Ninjin (Ginseng) Ginseng has been used in ethnopharmacology for more than 300 years. More than 28 kinds of ginsenosides and other active compounds have been isolated, and some have been shown to have biologic effects (Liu & Xiao, 1992).

Ginseng root saponin (GRS) has antistress effects. GRS, 10 mg/kg intraperitoneally, has been shown to suppress the damage to mitochondria and the decrease in noradrenaline, serotonin, and dopamine in the brain of mice placed in a hypobaric environment. This suppression disappeared in adrenalectomized mice.

Saiko (Bupleuri Radix) This plant is often used for psychiatric problems. One extract, 100 mg/kg saikogenin A, inhibited methamphetamine-induced hyperactivity and increased hexobarbital-induced sleep in mice (Shibata, 1970).

Engosaku (Corydalis Tuber) and *Oren (Coptidis Rhizoma)* *Engosaku* is important in *Gosei-ha,* one of two *Kampo* schools. It is used as a sedative and analgesic. Tetrahydropalmatine (THP), tetrahydroprotoberberine (THPB), and stepholidine (SPD) have been isolated (Fig. 2) (Guo-Zhang, 1987). THP has analgesic, sedative, and hypnotic effects. In addition, (-) THP inhibits amphetamine-induced motor activity. (-) THPBs were shown to inhibit dopamine D_1 and D_2 receptors by a receptor binding assay (Zhu, 1991). (-)SPD was found to be 18 times more potent than haloperidol in inhibiting dopamine D_1 receptors and 14 times less potent in inhibiting D_2 receptors.

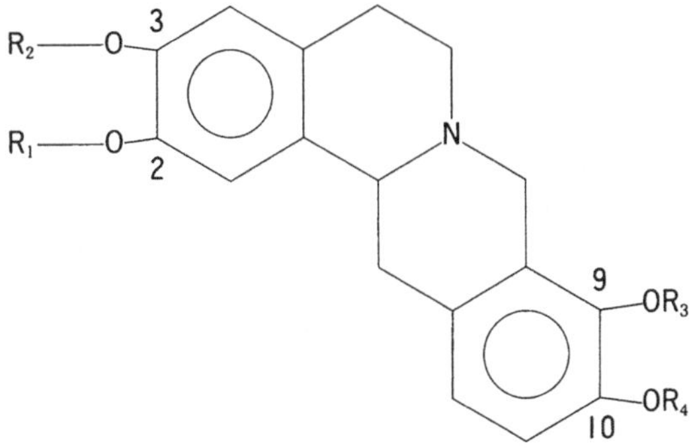

Compounds	R_1	R_2	R_3	R_4
THP [(+), (−)-]	CH_3	CH_3	CH_3	CH_3
THB	−CH_2−		CH_3	CH_3
(−)-SPD	H	CH_3	CH_3	H
(−)-scoulerine	H	CH_3	H	CH_3
(−)-corydalmine	CH_3	CH_3	CH_3	H
(±)-corypalmine	H	CH_3	CH_3	CH_3

Figure 2. Chemical structures of THP and its analogs. From Guo-Zhang, 1987, with permission.

The *Sho* of *Oren* is anxiety and upset stomach. *Oren* includes berberine and palmatine. Tetrahydroberberine and tetrahydropalmatine are thought to be formed by intestinal bacteria.

Daiou (Rhei Rhizoma) Daiou was once used to treat psychosis. A water extract of *Daiou* inhibited aggression by rats without olfactory organs and also inhibited methamphetamine-induced hyperactivity. The active compound is RG tannin, which was shown to inhibit noradrenaline, serotonin, and dopamine in the rat brain (Fujiwara et al., 1986).

Sanso-nin (Zizyphi Spinosi Semen) This plant was traditionally used to treat insomnia. The active compound, betulic acid, has anticholinergic and antihistaminergic effects (Shibata & Fukushima, 1975). This herb is known to inhibit caffeine-induced excitation and to prolong hexobarbital-induced sleep.

Koboku (Magnolia Cortex) Koboku has been used to induce sedation and analgesia and to treat psychiatric symptoms and stress ulcers. To date, only a few studies have been done. The ether extract is known to have a strong central depressant effect, and the water extract displays an inhibitory effect on excitation induced by dopamine agonists in mice (Watanabe, 1975).

TABLE 1.

Open Studies on the Efficacy of Herbal Medicines for Depressed States

Prescription	Diagnosis	Number	Improvement	Other drugs	Reference
Saiko-ka-ryukotsu-borei-to	Depression, neurosis	12	Effective	+	Kaneko et al. (1984)
Saiko-ka-ryukotsu-borei-to	Neurosis	23	>Moderate(17%) >Mild(78%)	+	Ohara et al. (1985)
Hange-kouboku-to	Neurosis	22	>Moderate(36%) >Mild(77%)	+	Ohara et al. (1985)
Yokukan-sann-ka-chinnpi-hange	Neurosis	20	>Moderate(15%) >Mild(70%)	+	Kanba and Asai(1991)
Saiboku-to	Neurosis	33	>Remarkable(9%) >Moderate(41%) >Mild(77%)	+	Murase et al. (1989)
Kami-kihi-to	Depression, neurosis	19	>Moderate(32%)	+	Ohara et al. (1992)
Kami-kihi-to	Neurosis	35	>Mild(57%)	+	Kudo et al. (1992)

Phase II Study of Herbal Formulas

A number of studies have been done on the efficacy of herbal medicine in Japan, as well as in China and Korea. Some of these are summarized in Table 1.

A particularly interesting herbal preparation frequently used in Japan is *Yokukannsan-ka-chinpi-hange* (YKCH) (Table 2). This formula contains nine plants and traditionally has been indicated for children's temper tantrums, irritable and explosive moods, and insomnia. The *Sho* of this formula is a patient with a poor constitution who is irritable and explosive or who has insomnia; palpitations in the umbilical region are often an indication of this preparation.

We studied the efficacy of YKCH in 31 patients with anxiety neurosis who had not adequately responded to psychotropics after eight weeks of administration (Kanba et al., 1991). We added YKCH, 7.5 g/day, to their regimen for four weeks. Their symptoms were rated according to the Hamilton Anxiety Scale at every visit. The average age of the patients was 56 ± 14 years. Figure 3 shows

TABLE   2.
Yokukan-San-Ka-Chinpi-Hange

Ingredients: 3.0 g tang-kuei,   4.0 g hoelen,   3.0 g gambir,   2.0 g bupleurum,   5.0 g pinellia,   3.0 g cnidium,   1.5 g licorice,   4.0 g atractylodes,   3.0 g citrus

Indications: Temper tantrums in children, irritable and explosive mood, insomnia, tics

Sho: Patients of poor constitution who are irritable and explosive or have insomnia. Palpitations in the umbilical region are often a good indicator.

---

the change in scores after the addition of YKCH. At the final evaluation, 3.2% of the patients showed remarkable improvement, 25.8% showed moderate improvement, and 38.7% exhibited mild improvement (Fig. 3). As for specific symptoms, insomnia, anxiety, tension, and depression showed relatively good improvement (Fig. 4). No side effects were reported. This study suggests that herbal medicine in combination with standard psychotropics may result in beneficial outcomes for therapy-resistant patients with neuroses.

Kami-kihi-to is a combination of 14 plants used for the treatment of neurosis, anemia,   and insomnia (Table 3).   Its traditional *Sho* is a patient of normal constitution with anxiety, irritability, insomnia, mild anemia, or low fever. A formulation containing *cinnamomi cortex* and *Glycyrrhitzae radix* is indicated for an imbalance of *Ki* distribution.

Recently, a multicenter open study was conducted to evaluate the efficacy of the formulation for various types of neurosis (Kudo et al., 1992). *Kami-kihi-to* was tried for eight weeks on 117 neurotic patients. Improvement was remarkable in 7.7%, moderate in 33.3 %, and mild in 57.3%. Anxiety neurosis and depressive neurosis responded to the formula better than did other types of neuroses. The symptoms of anxiety, tension, irritability, and neuroasthenia responded best. Fourteen percent of the patients experienced side effects, mostly gastrointestinal symptoms.

Saikoka-ryukotsu-borei-to, composed of 11 elements, can be effective for neurosis (Ohara et al., 1985), gynecologic problems, loss of energy, hypertension, arteriosclerosis, insomnia, cardiac neurosis, epilepsy, and Graves' disease (Table 4). The *Sho* of this formula is a patient with a strong constitution who has palpitations in the umbilical region, distention of the upper abdomen, and/or thoracocostal distress, as well as an irritable or depressive mood.

Hange-koboku-to is often prescribed for patients with neurosis with vertigo, paroxysmal palpitations, sensation of a foreign object in the throat, irritability, restlessness, and depression (Ohara et al., 1985). The formulation is composed of

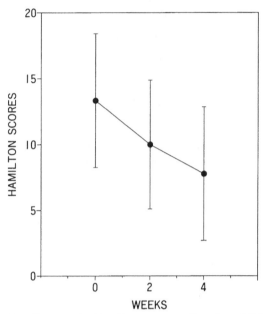

Figure 3. Changes in Hamilton scores after the addition of YKCH. For 31 patients with anxiety neuroses who were judged as not adequately responding to psychotropics after eight weeks of treatment, YKCH (7.5 g/day) was added for four weeks (Kanba et al., 1991). Symptoms were rated according to the Hamilton Anxiety Scale on every visit.

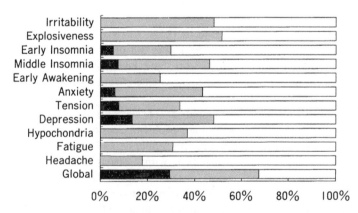

Figure 4. Final improvement in symptoms according to the following ratings: remarkable, moderate, mild, no change or worse.

TABLE 3.

Kami-Kihi-To

Ingredients: 2.0 g astragalus, 3.0 g zizyphus, 1.0 g licorice, 3.0 g ginseng, 3.0 g longan, 1.0 g saussurea, 3.0 g bupleurum, 3.0 g atracylodes, 2.0 g tang-kuei, 1.5 g ginger, 2.0 g gardenia, 3.0 g hoelen, 1.5 g polygala, 1.5 g jujube

Indications: Neurosis, anemia, insomnia

Sho: Patients of normal constitution who have anxiety, irritability, insomnia, mild anemia, or low fever.

five plants (Table 5). The traditional *Sho* indications are patients with a normal or poor constitution who have the sensation of a foreign object stuck in the throat, depressive mood, palpitations, insomnia, dyspnea, chest pain, vertigo, or distention beneath the heart. *Saiboku-to* is a similar formula.

KEIO UNIVERSITY HOSPITAL KAMPO CLINIC

Keio University Hospital opened a *Kampo* clinic in January 1993, which consists of an examination room equipped with thermography and an ultrasound scanner and a waiting room.

The staff of six physicians, with backgrounds in internal medicine, obstetrics/gynecology, anesthesiology, and psychiatry, sees, on average, eight new patients and 50 repeat patients every day.

Common problems observed in the clinic include psychosomatic symptoms, atopic dermatitis, allergic rhinitis, neuroses, irritable bowel syndrome, menopausal symptoms, insomnia, and chronic pain syndrome. These symptoms usually do not have an organic etiology nor do they respond to orthodox drugs. Some patients with difficult diseases, such as collagen disease, neoplasm, or chronic hepatitis, who have not achieved satisfactory results with modern medicine, come to the clinic for symptomatic relief. In these cases, in consultation with the patients' specialists, *Kampo* is prescribed in addition to the standard treatments.

FUTURE DIRECTIONS

The efficacy of several kinds of herbal formulas is now being evaluated in a randomized, double-blind, controlled study under the direction of the Ministry of Health and Welfare of Japan.

Since standard drugs and *Kampo* are often combined as a treatment strategy,

TABLE 4.

Saiko-Ka-Ryukotu-Borei-To

Ingredients: 5.0 g bupleurum, 2.5 g scute, 2.5 g dragon bone, 4.0 g pinellia, 2.5 g jujube, 2.5 g oyster shell, 3.0 g cinnamon, 2.5 g ginger, 1.0 g rhubarb, 3.0 g hoelen, 2.5 g ginseng

Indications: Neurosis, gynecologic problems, loss of energy, hypertension, arteriosclerosis, insomnia, cardiac neurosis, epilepsy, Basedow's disease

Sho: Patients of strong constitution who have palpitations in the umbilical region, distention of the upper abdomen, and/or thoracocostal distress, as well as an irritable or depressive mood.

TABLE 5.

Hange-Kouboku-To

Ingredients: 6.0 g pinellia, 3.0 g magnolia bark, 5.0 g hoelen, 2.0 g perilla, 4.0 g dried ginger

Indications: Neurosis with vertigo, paroxysmal palpitations, "hysteric ball," irritability, restlessness and depression

Sho: Patients of normal or poor constitution who have the sensation of a foreign object stuck in the throat, depressed mood, palpitations, insomnia, dyspnea, chest pain, vertigo, or distention beneath the heart

the benefits and potential side effects should be studied more extensively.

The pharmacologic study of mixtures of multiply acting compounds is to be carried on further. Such studies will reveal the mechanism of *kampo* medicine, and may lead to new psychotherapeutic agents with unique actions.

REFERENCES

Asai, M., Nakane, Y., Kanba, S. (1993): Diagnostic and therapeutic issues of atypical depression in Japan. *Eur. Psychiatry* **8**, 245-249.

Fujiwara, M., Iwasaki, K., Kurauchi, K., et al. (1986): The effect of RG-tannin on central nervous system (in Japanese). *Wakaniyakugakkaishi* **3**,322-323.

Guo-Zhang, J. (1987): (-)-Tetrajydropalmatine and its analogues as new dopamine receptor antagonists. *TIPS* **8**, 81-82.

Kanba, S., Mizuno, M., Yagi, G., Asai, M. (1991): Effects of *Tsumura Yoku-kann-sann-ka-chinnpi-hange* on neurosis (in Japanese). *Nikkei Medi.* **10**, 72-

73.

Kaneko, Y. (1994): Kampo medicine in psychiatry (in Japanese). *Rinsho-Seishin-Igaku* **13**, 19-32.

Kudo, Y., Mori, A., Asai, M., et al. (1992): Clinical evaluation of KAMIKIHI-TO (EK-49) in the treatment of psychoneurosis (in Japanese). *Rinsho-Iyaku* **8**, 203-221.

Liu, C., Xiao P.G. (1992): Recent advances on ginseng research in China. J. *Ethnopharmacol*. **36**, 27-38.

Murase, S., Kitamura, I., Murase, S., et al. (1989): Effects of *Tsumura Saibokuto* on anxiety neurosis (in Japanese). *Tumura Medical Information* **90**

Ohara, K., Fukazawa, H., Suzuki, Y., et al. (1985): The clinical effects of *Saiko-ka-ryukotsu-borei-to* and *Hange-koboku-to* on neurosis (in Japanese). *Sinyaku-to-Rinsho* **34**, 131-141.

Ohara, K., Kawaguchi, K., Tamefusa, N., et al. (1992): Efficacy of *Kami-Kihito* for insomnia in psychiatric disorders (in Japanese). *Tsumura Medical Information*, No. 113.

Shibata, M. (1970): Pharmacological studies on *Bupleurum falcatum* L (in Japanese). Yakugaku Zasshi **90**, 398-404.

Shibata, M., Fukushima, M. (1975): Acute toxicity and sedative action of Zizyphus seeds (in Japanese). *Yakugaku Zasshi* **95**, 465-469.

Terasawa, K. (1993): *Kampo: Japanese-Oriental Medicine. Insight from Clinical Cases*. Tokyo: Standard McIntyre.

Watanabe, K. (1975): Studies on the active principles of magnolia bark. Centrally acting muscle relaxant activity of magnolol and honokiol. Jpn. J. Pharmacol. **25**, 605-607.

Zhu, X-Z. (1991): Development of natural products as drugs acting on central nervous system. Mem. Inst. Oswaldo Cruz **86** (suppl II), 173-175.

2

Pharmacologic Studies of
Himbacine and Huperzine A:
Potential Use in Cholinergic Replacement Therapy*

M. McKinney and A.P. Kozikowski

Manipulations that would enhance levels of brain cholinergic tone are potential therapies for Alzheimer's disease and other diseases involving cholinergic degeneration. Protection of released acetylcholine with an acetylcholinesterase inhibitor is one well-known approach. Pharmacologic blockade of inhibitory presynaptic muscarinic receptors (autoreceptors) is another, less explored, possibility. We have been conducting studies on huperzine A, an acetylcholinesterase inhibitor, and on himbacine, a muscarinic antagonist, as agents that might be used to manipulate central cholinergic tone. Our pharmacologic studies have shown that rat hippocampal autoreceptors are largely of the M_4 category, with a possible contribution of the M_2 subtype. Using cloned human muscarinic receptors, himbacine has been shown to be a potent antagonist of the hm2 and hm4 receptors. Using in vitro *functional studies of brain muscarinic receptors, himbacine has been shown to bind to hippocampal presynaptic receptors at least 20-fold more potently than to postsynaptic muscarinic receptors coupled with phos-*

---

* Aspects of this review were presented at the Symposium on New Drug Development from Herbal Medicines in Neuropsychopharmacology, 19th CINP meeting, June 27-July 1, 1994, Washington, D.C.

Acknowledgments: Heptylphysostigmine was a gift of Dr. Paolo E. Lucchelli, Mediolanum Farmaceutici S.p.A., Milan, Italy. E2020 was a gift to Dr. Kozikowski. Dr. McKinney was assisted in the pharmacologic studies by J. H. Miller and P.J. Aagaard in his laboratory. We are grateful for the collaborations of the many associates of Dr. Kozikowski, including M. Malaska, W. Tuckmantel, A. Fauq, G. Campiani, and L.-Q. Sun. The work described was supported by grants AG09973, AG08031-02P1, and AG07591, and by the Mayo and Adler Foundations.

phoinositide turnover. We speculate that a therapy employing a combination of a muscarinic autoreceptor antagonist, such as himbacine, and an acetylcholinesterase inhibitor, such as huperzine A, may provide a highly selective and synergistic elevation of synaptic acetylcholine levels in cortex and hippocampus.

INTRODUCTION

The brain's cholinergic system has been the focus of many attempts at pharmacotherapy for Alzheimer's disease (AD) during the previous two decades. Generally, a variety of presynaptic and postsynaptic approaches to "cholinergic replacement" have resulted in limited efficacy, at best, and efforts in the current decade have largely been refocused on the possibilty of manipulating growth factor systems, upon which cholinergic systems are thought to depend. Now that it is known that several important neurotransmitter systems are actually at risk in AD, any approach that is limited to a single neurotransmitter system would not be expected to produce major beneficial effects in AD treatment. However, one might argue that manipulation of the cholinergic system is more feasible in the near term and that a partial effect is better than no treatment at all. With this point in mind, in previous reviews, we detailed the rationale for targeting the muscarinic receptors in AD pharmacotherapy (McKinney & Coyle, 1991;Kozikowski et al. 1992). Our viewpoint rests on the premise that, with five subtypes of this receptor expressed with anatomic heterogeneity in brain, with receptor subfamilies being coupled differentially to second messenger systems, and if selective ligands were to be developed, it might be possible to control central cholinergic tone pharmacologically. Early in the disease, or perhaps in some particular patients, there might be relatively selective cholinergic dysfunction, and these patients might respond in a substantive way to the appropriate drugs.

Elevation of synaptic acetylcholine is readily achievable using centrally acting acetylcholinesterase (AChE) inhibitors. In this regard, the only drug currently on the market for AD in the United States is tacrine, or tetrahydroaminoaceridine. This drug, while an effective AChE inhibitor, has a number of other sites of action and may cause hepatotoxicity in some patients (for a review of tacrine's pharmacological properties, see Freeman and Dawson, 1991). There are several other AChE inhibitors under development around the world, including E2020 in Japan and heptyl-physostigmine in Italy. Huperzine A has attracted our interest as a natural product and active principle in use in Chinese herbal medicine. The club moss, *Huperzia serrata*, is a component of a tea administered to elderly patients in China. This compound and the chemical cogener huperzine B were first isolated from the moss, identified, and shown to be potent AChE inhibitors by the Chinese (Jia-Sen *et al.*, 1986). Of particular interest to us is the selectivity of huperzine A for AChE versus butyrylcholinesterase (BuChE), which is at least two orders of magnitude, suggesting a high degree of selectivity for the putatively therapeutic target enzyme (Wang et al., 1986). The natural isomer of huperzine A is the (-) enantiomer, and the Chinese demonstrated that the mode of inhibition of AChE was mixed linear competitive, a type of noncompetitive inhibition (Wang et al., 1986). Huperzine A was first synthesized in the research laboratory by Kozikowski and colleagues in 1989 (Xia & Kozikowski, 1989); subsequently, an improved synthethic method was published (Campiani et al., 1993; Kozikowski et al., 1993). In a number of collaborative studies of the structure–activity relationships and preclinical pharmacology of huperzine A, this compound was confirmed to be a selective AChE inhibitor, to have little activity at non-AChE targets in a broad screen accomplished by NovaScreen, and to possess activity in behavioral studies (Interneuron, unpublished information).

MUSCARINIC AUTORECEPTORS AS TARGETS FOR PHARMACOTHERAPY

The muscarinic receptor family, currently with five subtypes, continues to be one of the most intensely studied members of the superfamily of G-protein coupled receptors, probably second in extent only to the closely related adrenergic receptors. Our interest has been in the selective coupling of members of the muscarinic family to second messenger systems, and utilization of conventional pharmacologic analyses to propose identities of those muscarinic receptors in brain (for a review, see McKinney, 1993). In the brain, the muscarinic receptors predominate in density over the nicotinic receptors, although both classes of proteins are certain to play important roles in cholinergic signal transduction. Many studies have supported a role for cholinergic positive neuromodulation of the cerebral cortex and hippocampus (for a review, see McKinney & Coyle, 1991), and muscarinic receptors are important for this. A simple view is that postsynaptic effects of acetylcholine in these regions are mediated mainly by M_1, M_3, and M_4 receptors, which form the bulk of the brain muscarinic receptor population, while some muscarinic receptors reside on the terminals of the cholinergic afferents. These presynaptic muscarinic receptors have been shown, both *in vitro* and *in vivo*, to mediate a feedback inhibition of acetylcholine release (for a recent example in human tissue, see Feuerstein et al., 1992). Most recently, direct evidence *in vivo* using microdialysis techniques in rodents has been obtained, demonstrating that these autoreceptors are major sites of control of release of the neurotransmitter (Stillman et al., 1993).

Pharmacologic studies of the cortical and hippocampal presynaptic muscarinic receptors have, on the one hand, suggested that they are made up of M_2

receptors (Richards, 1990), but, on the other hand, that they may be mainly M_4 receptors (McKinney et al., 1993). The data in each of these cited studies are quite strong in support of each subtype, and methodological differences may explain the conflicting results. Probably, both receptors are used as autoreceptors, and the conditions of assay may reveal one class or the other preferentially (e.g., use of chemical or electrical depolarization). In support of autoreceptor roles for both subtypes is the finding that the agonist efficacy profile for the hippocampal autoreceptor is mixed M_2/M_4 (McKinney et al., 1993), and that both m2 and m4 mRNAs have been localized in close association with basal forebrain cholinergic neurons that project to the hippocampus (Vilaro et al., 1993). The M_2 and M_4 receptors are very similar pharmacologically; most antagonists do not differentiate between them and only certain partial agonists display relatively subtle differences in rank orders of intrinsic efficacy (McKinney et al., 1991a). Thus, if both subtypes are functional autoreceptors, a presynaptic autoreceptor blocker may not need to be absolutely selective between these subtypes.

If elevation of the levels of synaptic acetylcholine is to be considered a desirable approach to cholinergic "replacement" therapy, then this could in theory be achieved, not only by using an AChE inhibitor, but also by inhibition of the autoreceptor. This is not a new idea: Crews and his colleagues (Crews et al., 1986), and Potter and his colleagues (Mash et al., 1985) suggested this some years ago. While most industrial efforts at developing new cholinergic drugs have focused on less toxic AChE inhibitors or on M_1 agonists, it is only recently that some attention is being given to the possibility to developing an autoreceptor antagonist. Prominently, Quirion and his associates have been proponents of the development of antagonists selective for the muscarinic autoreceptors (Quirion et al.,1989), and have had some considerable success (Doods et al., 1993). While the possible improvement in memory function by administration of a muscarinic antagonist seems counterintuitive, the neurobiology of muscarinic receptor subtypes suggests that it is possible. Using calculations involving the coupling efficiencies of pre- and postsynaptic systems in cortex/hippocampus, in a simplified and ideal cholinergic synapse, this antagonist would be predicted to be behaviorally effective if it were 44-fold or more selective for the autoreceptor, and, if it is to have an acceptable therapeutic window, this selectivity should probably be at least 100-fold. The M_2 receptor could be considered the more desirable central target, as it seems that it is more likely to be largely devoted to the autoreceptor role, while the M_4 receptor is almost as prominent in cortex and hippocampus as is the M_1 receptor. Since only a small minority of muscarinic receptors are located presynaptically, the bulk of M_4 receptors must be postsynaptic. Whether the blockade of postsynaptic M_4 receptors would enhance or degrade the positive influence of cholinergic input to these regions is completely unknown. From an alternative perspective, the M_4 receptor might be more suitable as a target for an autoreceptor antagonist, because such a drug should not affect the M_2 muscarinic receptors located in cardiac tissue. At any rate, currently there are no muscarinic antagonists that have a 100-fold, or even the minimal 44-fold, level of selectivity for the M_2/M_4 subtypes, as compared with the M_1 receptor.

Despite the limitations of the currently available agents, there are already indications that enhancement of learning and memory will occur with presynaptic autoreceptor blockade. Packard and colleagues were first to show that improvement in memory behavior in rats would result from administration of an M_2-selective agent, AF-DX 116 (Packard et al., 1990). This antagonist has only modest M_2 potency and is only about 5- to 10- fold selective for the M_2 receptor over the M_1 receptor. The effect of AF-DX 116 on a memory task was confirmed in mice (Baratti et al., 1993). Additionally, this latter group showed that a centrally acting AChE inhibitor and AF-DX 116 synergistically enhanced memory performance. This finding suggests that combination cholinergic replacement might be much more effective in AD, as we and others have speculated (Feuerstein et al., 1992; McKinney & Coyle, 1991; Baratti et al., 1993).

STUDIES OF THE ACETYLCHOLINESTERASE INHIBITOR HUPERZINE A

Lineweaver-Burke analysis of the stereoisomers of huperzine A indicated that the natural substance, (-)-huperzine A, was over 40-fold more potent that (+)-huperzine for inhibition of rat cortical AChE (McKinney et al., 1991b). In these experiments, we confirmed the Chinese finding that (-) huperzine A was a mixed linear competitive inhibitor of AChE (Wang et al., 1986) and found, additionally, that (+) huperzine A displayed the same inhibition kinetics. More recently, we conducted a study comparing several anticholinesterases for selectivity in inhibiting AChE (rat cortical) versus BuChE (rat serum) *in vitro*; (+/-)-huperzine A was almost 500-fold selective for the former enzyme (Table I). In the same study, E2020 was found to be the next most selective agent (172-fold), while THA, physostimine, and heptyl-physostigmine were essentially nonselective (Table I). The data in Table I were obtained under conditions in which the [substrate]/K_m values for AChE and BuChE were similar, making direct comparisons of the IC_{50} values meaningful. Another indication of desirable selectivity in an AChE inhibitor is a lack of potency in blocking muscarinic receptors. As Table 2 shows, (+/-) huperzine A at concentrations up to 100 μM did not inhibit M_1 or M_2 muscarinic receptor binding, while the other AChE inhibitors tested bound with modest potencies to these subtypes.

Numerous analogs of huperzine A were synthesized by Dr. Kozikowski and colleagues in a study of its pharmacophoric elements; none of these compounds

TABLE 1.

Potencies and Selectivities for Inhibition of Acetylcholinesterase (AChE) and Pseudocholinesterase (ChE) by Five Anticholinesterase Drugs*

Drug	AChE IC_{50} (μM) (n)	ChE IC_{50} (μM) (n)	Selectivity ratio
(+/-) Huperzine A	0.056 +/- 0.004 (6)	26 +/- 0.02 (5)	464
E2020	0.018 +/- 0.001 (6)	3.1 +/- 0.7 (4)	172
Physostigmine	0.022 +/- 0.003 (6)	0.077 +/- 0.011 (5)	3.5
Heptyl-physostigmine	0.44 +/- 0.033 (4)	0.172 +/- 0.031 (4)	0.4
THA	0.139 +/- 0.013 (6)	0.229 +/- 0.046 (4)	1.6

* Rat cortical AChE was assayed as described (McKinney et al., 1991b). Rat serum BuChE was assayed with a kit from Sigma Chemical Company (St. Louis). The ratios of [substrate]/K_m in the two assays were similar; thus the IC_{50} values are directly comparable

TABLE 2.

Interactions of anticholinesterases with muscarinic receptors*

Drug receptor	M_1 Muscarinic receptor IC_{50} (μM)	M_2 Muscarinic receptor IC_{50} (μM)
(+/-) Huperzine A	> 100	> 100
E2020	3.44 +/- 0.3	2.54 +/- 0.11
Physostigmine	100 +/- 2.4	100 +/- 6.5
Heptyl-physostigmine	12.7 +/- 0.8	14.8 +/- 0.23
THA	5.6 +/- 0.2	4.46 +/- 0.02

* Radioligand binding was performed with hml human muscarinic receptors (M_1) transfected into CHO cells and with rat brain stem (M_2 receptors). The concentration of radioligand was comparable in the two assays; thus the IC_{50} values are directly comparable.

were as potent as the parent compound for the inhibition of AChE (data not shown). Similarly, in a study of a series of huperzine A analogs by the Chinese group, none were described that were as potent as (-) huperzine A (Tang et al., 1994). Thus, to date, the most potent AChE inhibitor incorporating the huperzine skeleton is the parent structure, (-) huperzine A. While this alkaloid is not the most potent AChE inhibitor known, the Chinese report that it is efficacious in demented patients and displays no toxic side effects (Zhang et al., 1991;Tang et al., 1989). Thus, if new AChE inhibitors continue to be considered a viable approach to AD therapy, huperzine A will be an outstanding candidate.

DEVELOPMENT OF PRESYNAPTIC ANTAGONISTS AND STUDIES OF HIMBACINE

Along the lines of developing a selective inhibitor for the presynaptic muscarinic autoreceptor, medicinal chemistry and pharmacology have been combined by Quirion and associates to improve on the properties of AF-DX 116, to produce agents like AQ-RA741. Subsequent work by this group of investigators was conducted to develop M_2 antagonists with improved selectivity and brain penetration, resulting in such compounds as BIBN 99 (Doods et al., 1993).

Our own efforts have been more limited and directed at the alkaloid himbacine. Himbacine is a member of a family of alkaloids isolated from the bark of trees of the *Galbulimima* species in Australia (Richie & Taylor, 1967) and is known to be a potent antimuscarinic. There have been numerous reports of the selectivity of himbacine for cardiac receptors (Anwar-ul et al., 1986; Gilani & Cobbin, 1987; Choo et al., 1988; Eglen et al., 1988; Lazareno & Roberts, 1989; Darroch et al., 1990). In a study of a number of naturally occurring analogs of himbacine, its cardioselectivty was shown to depend in part on the existence of a methylated nitrogen (as evidenced in the loss of selectivity with the analog himbeline), while himbacine's M_2 potency depends in part on the correct orientation of the other methyl substituent in the side group (as is evidenced by the loss of M_2 selectivity with *N*-methyl-himandravine) (Darroch et al., 1990). The double bond in the bridge is also important for M_2 selectivity (Darroch et al., 1990). Himbacine's M_2 selectivity was confirmed using cloned human muscarinic receptors (Dorje et al., 1991; Miller et al., 1992). Since himbacine was reported to be selective for the M_2 muscarinic receptor, and because it is thought that this subtype serves as an autoreceptor for the control of acetylcholine release, we were interested in the potential for himbacine to enhance synaptic levels of acetylcholine by blockade of presynaptic muscarinic receptors, perhaps combined with the administration of an anticholinesterase such as huperzine A.

Using cloned human muscarinic receptors, we showed that himbacine bound potently to both hm2 and hm4 receptors, and was 10- to 50-fold less potent at hml, hm3, or hm5 subtypes (Miller et al., 1992). These studies also showed that himbacine was about 20-fold more potent in hippocampal preparations for blocking presynaptic receptors as compared with putative postsynaptic muscarinic receptors. A number of analogs of himbacine were synthesized to evaluate major regions of the molecule important for M_2 selectivity. Upon replacing the himbacine tricyclic moiety with dihydroanthracene or dibenzosuberyl rings, potencies for M_1 and M_2 receptors increased dramatically but M_2 selectivity was reduced or eliminated (Malaska et al., 1993). In further work, we have shown that the carbonyl functionality in the tricycle is important in the M_2 selectivity of himbacine; for example, opening this ring to form a diol, or substituting an ether oxygen in the ring in place of the carbonyl oxygen results in the loss of most of the M_2 selectivity of himbacine (Malaska et al., 1995).

CONCLUSION

While one can argue convincingly that the efficacious treatment of Alzheimer's disease will require the development of completely novel agents that intercede in the mechanism of neurodegeneration, this type of approach is hindered by some uncertainty as to the true etiology of the disease. On the other hand, loss of cholinergic projections is virtually an invariant finding in the brains of Alzheimer's patients. If any aspect of learning or memory is degraded by the loss of brain acetylcholine, then some efficacy might result in the selective potentiation of this neurotransmitter. Unfortunately, selective targeting of the regions of the brain experiencing the loss of acetylcholine is limited by the lack of selective cholinomimetics. However, this chapter has summarized the potential for two novel alkaloids, huperzine A and himbacine, to be agents that could, in theory, synergistically enhance cholinergic tone in the cortex and hippocampus.

REFERENCES

Anwar-ul, S., Gilani, H., Cobbin, L.B. (1986): The cardio-selectivity of himbacine: A muscarine receptor antagonist. *Naunyn-Schmied. Arch. Pharmacol.* **332**, 16-20.

Baratti, C.M., Opezzo, J.W., Kopf, S.R. (1993): Facilitation of memory storage by the acetylcholine M_2 muscarinic receptor antagonist AF-DX 116. *Behav. Neur. Biol.* **60**, 69-74.

Campiani, G., Sun, L.-Q., Kozikowski, A.P., et al. (1993): A palladium-catalyzed route to huperzine A and its analogues and their anticholinesterase activity. *J. Org. Chem.* **58**, 7660-7669.

Choo, L.K., Mitchelson, F., Napier, P. (1988): Differences in antagonist affinities at muscarinic receptors in chick and guinea-pig. *J. Auton. Pharmacol.* **8**, 259-266.

Crews, F.T., Meyer, E.M., Gonzales, R.A., et al. (1986): Presynaptic and postsynaptic approaches to enhancing central cholinergic neurotransmission. In: T. Crook, R.T. Bartus, S. Ferris, S. Gershon (Eds.), *Treatment Development Strategies for Alzheimer's Disease*, pp.335-419. Madison,Conn.: Mark Powley Associates.

Darroch, S.A., Taylor, W.C., Choo, L.K., Michelson, F. (1990): Structure-activity relationships for some Galbulimima alkaloids related to himbacine. *Euro. J. Pharmacol.*, **182**, 131-136.

Doods, H.N., Quirion, R., Mihm, G., et al. (1993): Therapeutic potential of CNS-active M_2 antagonists: novel structures and pharmacology. *Life Sci.* **52**, 497-503.

Dorje, F., Wess, J., Lambrecht, G., et al. (1991): Antagonist binding profiles of five cloned human muscarinic receptor subtypes. *J.Pharmacol. Exp. Ther.* **256**, 272-733.

Eglen, R.M., Montgomery, W.W., Dainty, I.A., et al. (1988): The interaction of methoctramine and himbacine at atrial, smooth muscle and endothelial muscarinic receptors in vitro. *Br. J. Pharmacol.* **95**, 1031-1038.

Feuerstein, T.J., Lehmann, J., Sauermann. W., et al. (1992) : The autoinhibitory feedback control of acetylcholine release in human neocortex tissue. *Brain Res.* **572**, 64-71.

Freeman, S.E., Dawson, R.M. (1991): Tacrine: A pharmacological review. *Prog. Neurobiol.* **36**, 257-277.

Gilani, S.A., Cobbin, L.B. (1987): Interaction of himbacine with carbachol at muscarinic receptors of heart and smooth muscle. *Arch. Int. Pharmacodyn.* **290**, 46-53.

Jia-Sen, L., Chao-Mei, Y., Zhou, Y. -Z., et al. (1986): Study on the chemistry of huperzine A and B. *Acta Chim. Sin.* **44**, 1035-1040.

Kozikowski, A.P., Campiani, G., Aagaard, P.J., McKinney, M. (1993): An improved synthetic route to huperzine A: new analogues and their inhibition of acetylcholinesterase. *J. Chem. Soc. Chem. Commun.* **10**, 860-861.

Kozikowski, A.P., Fauq, A.H., Miller, J.H., McKinney, M. (1992): Alzheimer's therapy:An approach to novel muscarinic ligands based upon the naturally occurring alkaloid himbacine. *Bio-Org. Med. Chem. Lett.* **2**, 797-802.

Lazareno, S., Roberts, F.F. (1989): Functional and binding studies with muscarinic M_2-subtype selective antagonists. *Br. J. Pharmacol.* **98**, 309-317.

Malaska, M. J., Fauq, A.H., Kozikowski, A.P., et al. (1993): Simplified analogs of himbacine displaying potent binding affinity for muscarinic receptors. *Bio.-org. Med. Chem. Lett.* **3**, 1247-1252.

Malaska, M.J., Fauq, A.H., Kozikowski, A.P., et al. (1995): Chemical modification of ring C of himbacine: Discovery of a pharmacophoric element for M_2-selectivity. *Bio.-Org. Med. Chem. Lett.*, **5**, 61 − 66.

Mash, D.C., Flynn, D.D., Potter, L.T. (1985): Loss of M_2 muscarine receptors in the cerebral cortex in Alzheimer's disease and experimental cholinergic denervation. *Science* **228**, 1115-1117.

McKinney, M. (1993): Muscarinic receptor subtype-specific coupling to second messengers in neuronal systems. *Prog. Brain Res.* **98**. 333-340.

McKinney, M., Coyle, J.T. (1991): The potential for muscarinic receptor subtype-specific pharmacotherapy for Alzheimer's disease. *Mayo Clin. Proc.* **66**, 1225-1237.

McKinney, M., Miller, J.H., Aagaard, P.J. (1993): Pharmacological characterization of the rat hippocampal muscarinic autoreceptor *J. Pharmacol. Exp. Ther*. **264**, 74-78.

McKinney, M., Miller, J.H., Gibson. J.H., et al. (1991a): Interactions of agonists with M_2 and M_4 muscarinic receptor subtypes mediating cyclic AMP inhibition. *Mol. Pharmacol*. **40**, 1014-1022.

McKinney, M. Miller, J.H., Yamada, F., et al. (1991b): Potencies and stereoselectivities of enantiomers of huperzine A for inhibition of rat cortical acetylcholinesterase. *Eur. J Pharmacol*. **203**, 303-305.

Miller, J.H., Aagaard, P.J., Gibson, V.A., McKinney, M. (1992): Binding and functional selectivity of himbacine for cloned and neuronal muscarinic receptors. *J. Pharmacol. Exp. Ther*. **263**, 663-667.

Packard, M.G., Regenold, W., Quirion, R., White, N.M. (1990): Post-training injection of the acetylcholine M_2 receptor antagonist AF-DX 116 improves memory. *Brain Res*. **524**, 72-76.

Quirion, R. Aubert, I., Lapchak, P.A., et al. (1989): Muscarinic receptor subtypes in human neurodegenerative disorders: Focus on Alzheimer's disease. *Trends Pharmacol. Sci. Suppl.*, 80-84.

Richards, M.H. (1990): Rat hippocampal muscarinic autoreceptors are similar to the M_2 (cardiac) subtype: comparison with hippocampal M_1, atrial M_2, and ileal M_3 receptors. *Br. J. Pharmacol*. **99**, 753-761.

Richie, E., Taylor, W.C. (1967): The *Galbulimima* alkaloids, In: R.H.F. Manske (Ed.), *The Alkaloids IX*, pp. 529-543. New York: Academic Press.

Stillman, M.J., Shukitt-Hale, B., Kong, R.M., et al. (1993): Elevation of hippocampal extracellular acetylcholine levels by methoctramine. *Brain Res. Bull*. **32**, 385-389.

Tang, X.-C., Desarno, P., Sugaya, K., et al. (1989): Effect of huperzine A, a new cholinesterase inhibitor, on the central cholinergic system of the rat. *J. Neurosci. Res*., **24**, 276-285.

Tang, X.-C., Xu H, Feng, J., et al. (1994): Effect of cholinesterase inhibition in vitro by huperzine analogs. *Acta Pharmacol. Sin*. **15**, 107-110.

Vilaro, M. T., Mengod, G., Palacios, J.M. (1993): Advances and limitations of the molecular neuroanatomy of cholinergic receptors: The example of multiple muscarinic receptors. *Prog. Brain. Res*. **98**, 95-101.

Wang, Y.-E., Yue, D.-X., Tang, X.-C. (1986): Anti-cholinesterase activity of huperzine A. *Acta Pharmacol. Sin*. **7**, 110-113.

Xia, Y., Kozikowski, A.P. (1989): A practical synthesis of the Chinese "nootropic" agent huperzine A: A possible lead in the treatment of Alzheimer's disease. *J. Am. Chem. Soc*. **111**, 4116.

Zhang, R.W., Tang, X.-C., Han, Y.Y., et al. (1991): Drug evaluation of huperzine A in the treatment of senile memory disorders. *Acta Pharmaco. Sin*. **12**, 250-252.

3

Neuropharmacologic Activity of Constituents Isolated from Chinese Medicinal Plants*

X. C. Tang

The chemical investigation of Chinese medicinal plants has been a favorite area of research, leading to the isolation of hundreds of constituents and the elucidation of the structures of many novel and complex molecules at the Shanghai Institute of Materia Medica. Distinct structural classes of constituents were tested at different levels pharmacologically. l-Curine was first found in a Chinese plant; its quaternary salt had significant neuromuscular blocking activity. Many alkaloids isolated from Chinese Aconitum had promising analgesic activity. They belonged to nonnarcotic class of analgesia. These studies agree very well with Aconitum's therapeutic properties in Chinese traditional medicine. Five naturally occurring cholinesterase (ChE) inhibitors have been found in Chinese medicinal plants. Huperzine A so far is the most potent selective acetylcholinesterase (AChE) inhibitor, and is a promising candidate for clinical development for the treatment of cholinergic-related neurodegenerative disorders.

INTRODUCTION

Today, when pure compounds are often preferred as drugs, some of the most valuable compounds are still isolated from plants rather than prepared synthetically. Therefore, bioactive compounds of natural origin are important targets of chemists, and a great deal of attention has been given to the therapeutic use of

---

* Presented at the Symposium on New Drug Development from Herbal Medicines in Neuropsychopharmacology of the 19th CINP Congress, June 27–July 1, 1994, Washington, D.C.

herbal remedies.

Traditional medicine and remedies have been practiced and used since ancient times in the fight against disease in China. Many Chinese still depend on the Chinese system of medicine, and although mineral and animal products are used to some extent, most part of indigenous drugs are from plants. Thousands of plants have proved to be valuable based on long-term observation and clinical trials. It is clear that owing to China's rich natural resources and the achievements of Chinese ancient medical practice, there is considerable potential for fruitful ethnopharmacologic studies, and herbal medicine is recognized as the most efficient way to develop new or prototype drugs in China.

Since the 1950s, persistent efforts have been made toward developing new drugs from Chinese medicinal plants at this Institute. Over 400 constituents so far have been isolated from plants. Some constituents have known structures, but unknown pharmacologic activities; some are poorly recognized as to their pharmacologic activities; and some have novel chemical structures. In this chapter, a number of natural constituents exhibiting neuropharmacologic activities are discussed.

CONSTITUENT
NEUROMUSCULAR BLOCKING ACTIVITY

Cyclea barbata and *Cyclea hainanensis* are indigenous plants that are widely available on China's Hai-nan Island. *C barbata* has been reported to cure laryngitis, abdominal pain, toothache, trauma, and fractures (Tang et al., 1980b). Despite its long period of use, there was no study to verify its pharmacologic effects until the 1970s. *C barbata* and *C hainanensis* were selected for study on the basis of their total alkaloid presenting muscle-relaxing activity in preliminary experiments. Six alkaloids (*l*-curine. *dl*-curine, 4"-*o*-methyl-*d*-curine, homoaromoline, *d*-tetrandrine, and *d*-isochondrodendrine) were identified on the basis of spectroscopic and chemical evidence (Shanghai Institute of Materia Medica, 1979). Subsequently, *l*-curine was also isolated from *C hypoglauca* (Schauer) Diels and *Cissampelos pareria* Linn collected in the Guang-Xi and Yun-Nan provinces of China. In rabbits, the head-drop test showed that the quaternary salt of these alkaloids had relaxing effects on neck muscles. *o,o*-Dimethyl derivatives of curine were more potent than their parent quaternary compounds, which emphasized the importance of steric factors in this activity (Table 1).

Extensive pharmacologic testing showed *o,o*-dimethyl *l*-curine dimethochloride (*l*-DCD) to be the most effective relaxant as determined in mice, rats, rabbits, cats, and dogs. The effective dose varied from 0.04 to 0.16 mg/kg given intravenously; *l*-DCD was about 0.5 to four times more active than *d*-tubocurarine (*d*-tc) (Tang et al., 1980a, 1980b). The rate of decline of the

TABLE 1.

Neuromuscular-Blocking Activity of Curine and Its Derivatives.

Compounds	R_1	R_2	R_3	R_4	Configuration A	Configuration B	Relative potency*
1	H	H	Me	Me	R	R	
2	H	H	(Me)$_2$	(Me)$_2$	R	R	1.77
3	Me	Me	(Me)$_2$	(Me)$_2$	R	R	2.68
4	H	Me	Me	Me	S	S	
5	H	Me	(Me)$_2$	(Me)$_2$	S	S	0.69
6	Me	Me	(Me)$_2$	(Me)$_2$	S	S	0.84
7	H	H	Me	Me	R	R	
					S	S	
8	H	H	(Me)$_2$	(Me)$_2$	R	R	1.45
					S	S	
9	Me	Me	(Me)$_2$	(Me)$_2$	R	R	1.94
					S	S	
10	H	H	(Me)$_2$	Me	S	R	1.00
				H			

* Rabbit head-drop test. Compounds: (1) *l*-curine; (2) *l*-curine dimethochloride; (3) dimethyl *l*-curine dimethochloride; (4) 4″-*o*-methyl-*d*-curine; (5) 4″-*o*-methyl-*d*-curine dimethochloride; (6) dimethyl 4″-*o*-methyl-*d*-curine dimethochloride; (7) *dl*-curine; (8) *dl*-curine dimethochloride; (9) dimethyl *dl*-curine dimethochloride; (10) *d*-tubocurarine.

neuromuscular-blocking activity was dose dependent, decreasing with increasing dose (Huang et al., 1983). The neuromuscular-blocking activity of *l*-DCD was readily reversed by neostigmine, antagonized by saxamethonium, and potentiated by *d*-tc. Tetanus was poorly sustained during *l*-DCD block, and post-tetanic potentiation occurred (Tang et al., 1980b). *l*-DCD abolished the response of the chick's biventer cervicis muscle to acetylcholine (ACh) after its indirectly elicited maximal twitches were blocked, and reduced the amplitude of end-plate potential and miniature end-plate potential in the rat's phrenic nerve-diaphragm preparation. The membrane potential of diaphragm muscle fibers was not altered by *l*-DCD (Yang and Linn, 1981).

In view of these results, it was concluded that *l*-DCD is a nondepolarizing relaxant. It has a postsynaptic blocking effect at the neuromuscular junction. Full relaxation of muscle with *l*-DCD was achieved in humans with doses in the range of 0.3 to 0.5 mg/kg. The onset time was 1 to 3 minutes while the recovery time was about 30 to 50 minutes for a 0.3 mg/kg dose. Ideal intubate conditions could be achieved with 0.4 to 0.5 mg/kg (Wang, 1981b). The ganglion blocking activity and histamine-releasing property of *l*-DCD were weaker than with *d*-tc. It is looked upon as fulfilling the requirements for a nondepolarizing neuromuscular-blocking agent with an intermediate duration of action.

ACTIVE ALKALOIDS OF CHINESE ACONITUM

The root of *Aconitum* is a well-known plant that has been used since ancient times in Chinese traditional medicine. Some 170 *Aconitum* species are found in China, chiefly in the southwestern and northwestern provinces. Forty-four *Aconitum* species have been recorded as being used medicinally for various ailments (Wang, 1981a).

Chinese *Aconitum* has been used frequently as a component of numerous prescriptions, for relieving colds, rheumatoid arthritis, and pain and swelling induced by trauma and fracture, as well as an anodyne and a cardiotonic. A broad-based screening of *Aconitum* for a wide range of biologic activities is being continued in China. To date, about 20 *Aconitum* species have been subjected to scientific testing and experimentation, and over 170 alkaloids isolated (Wang, 1981a). As early as the 1950s, phytochemists in this Institute began to study the active principles of Chinese *Aconitum*; 102 alkaloids were isolated from 16 species, of which 46 were new alkaloids. Diterpenoid alkaloid aconitine is the principal alkaloid in most *Aconitum* species, but other related alkaloids are normally present as well (Fig. 1). Pharmacologic studies from this Institute showed that most of the alkaloids exhibited significant analgesic and local anesthetic activities (Table 2). Some alkaloids were found to possess antithermic effects in normothermic and pyrexial rodents (Lin et al., 1987; Liu et al., 1987), as well as anti-inflammatory effects assayed with several animal inflammatory models (Tang et al., 1984; Lin et al., 1987). Yunaconitine showed immunomodulating action in addition to analgesic and anti-inflammatory activities (Li et al., 1987b). *Guan-Fu* base A had a significant anti-arrhythmic effect (Chen et al., 1983). Some alkaloids, such as 3-acetylaconitine (AAC), bulleyaconitine A (BUL), and lappaconitine (LA), had completed preclinical and clinical trials, and have been introduced for the treatment of several kinds of chronic pain, rheumatoid arthritis, and so on.

The analgesic actions of AAC, BUL, LA, and *N*-deacetyllappaconitine (DLP)

	R_1	R_2	R_3	R_4
Aconitine	CH_3CH_2	OH	H	OH
3-acetylaconitine	CH_3CH_2	OAc	H	OH
Nagarine	CH_3CH_2	OH	OH	OH
Penduline	CH_3CH_2	H	H	H
Buiwutine	CH_3	OH	OH	OH

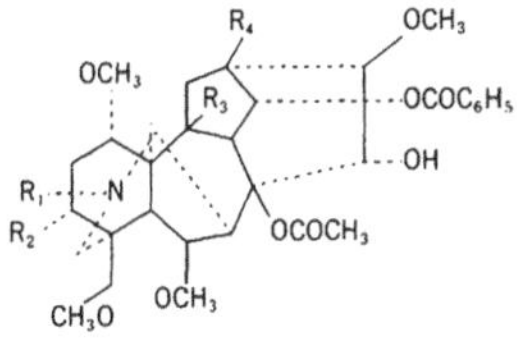

Bulleyaconitine A   R = H

Yunaconitine   R = OH

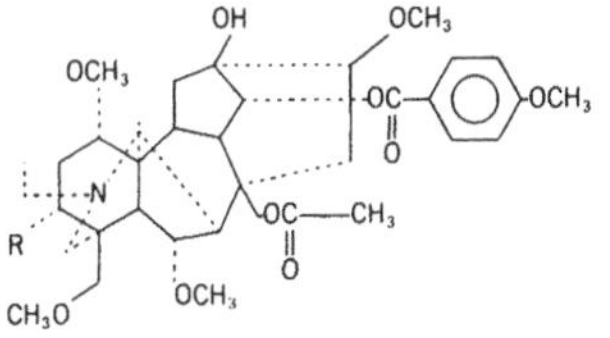

	R_1	R_2	R_3	R_4
Lappaconitine	H	OH	H	$COCH_3$
Ranaconitine	OH	OH	H	$COCH_3$
Deacetylranaconitine	OH	OH	H	H
Deacetylfinaconitine	OH	OH	OH	H
Deacetyllappaconitine	H	OH	H	H

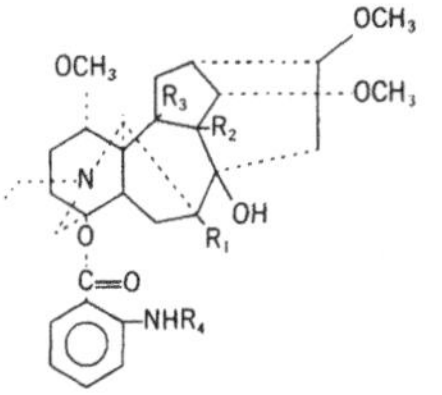

Figure 1. Chemical structures of alkaloids isolated from Chinese *Aconitum* species.

have been investigated in detail by using such methods as acetic acid-induced writhing, a hot plate, formaldehyde-elicited continuous pain stimuli in mice, and rat tail-flick response to light irradiation. The relative analgesic effect of BUL was found to be 1.8 to 3.25, 15.3 to 65.5, and 1208 to 7195 times as potent as AAC, morphine, and aspirin respectively (Tang et al., 1986b). The analgesic effects of BUL and AAC lasted longer than that of morphine. AAC, LA, or DLA potentiated the analgesia of morphine, which was reversed by naloxone but did not affect the analgesia induced by AAC, LA, or DLA. Analgesia mediated by AAC, BUL, or LA was eliminated by intraperitoneal injection of reserpine three hours prior to AAC, BUL or LA, and was enhanced by elevation of brain 5-HT or norepinephrine level (Tang et al., 1986a; Lu et al., 1988; Guo & Tang, 1990a). AAC-, BUL-, or LA-induced analgesia was also found to be attenuated or augmented by the administration of chemicals related to brain monoamines (Table 3). The results showed that the central catecholaminergic and serotoninergic systems are involved in the modulation of analgesia induced by AAC, BUL, or LA. Electrolytic or kainic acid lesion experiments showed that superspinal

TABLE 2.

Pharmacologic Activities of Alkaloids from Chinese *Aconitum* in Mice

Alkaloids	Analgesic ED_{50} dose (mg/kg, SC)		Sciatic nerve block	Acute LD_{50}
	Hot plate	HAc,writing	IC_{50}, %	(mg/kg, SC)
Aconitine	0.13	0.062	0.0074	0.31
3-acetylaconitine*	0.16	0.156	0.0025	1.4
Lappaconitine	5.6(+)	3.5	0.04	11.7
Ranaconitine		4.2	0.1	9.0
Yunaconitine	0.042	0.039		0.37
Bulleyaconitine A*	0.087	0.048	0.0029	0.92
N-deacetylaconitine	8.6	2.3	0.076	36.4
N-deacetylranaconitine*		8.6	0.1	27.5
N-deacetylfinaconitine*		8.6	0.102	> 50
Avadharidine		52.5	1.0(−)	45.9
Lycoctonine		144	1.0(−)	>500
Penduline*	0.94	0.89	0.105	3.9
Mesaconitine	0.069	0.041	0.0042	0.157
Buiwutine*	0.154	0.06	0.05(−)	0.39
Songoline	100(−)		17.4	>300
Neoline	150(−)		20(−)	>400
Denudatine	50(−)		20(−)	207
Deoxyaconitine	0.9	0.48	0.011	2.8
Hypaconitine	0.65	0.31	0.016	2.8
Nagarine*		0.14	0.01(−)	1.22
Morphine	5.7	0.8		
Aspirin	626	195		
Cocaine			0.25	

(+) Effective dose.   (−) Ineffective dose.   *New alkaloid.

sites, especially the peri aqueductal gray (PAG) and nucleus raphe magnus, are involved in LA- and DLA-induced analgesia (Guo & Tang, 1990b). Microinjection of $CaCl_2$ into the PAG area reduced LA-induced analgesia, indicating that LA can produce analgisia, possibly through a decrease in cellular calcium availability, and PAG may be involved in the Ca^{2+} antagonistic effect on LA analgesia (Guo & Tang, 1989).

Contrasting with the central analgesic effect of opiates, AAC, BUL, or LA did not cause tolerance when repeatedly injected in mice. No abstinence syndrome was seen after sudden AAC, BUL, or LA withdrawal, or when challenged with nalorphine. No physical dependence on AAC, BUL, or LA has been shown in rats and monkeys that developed physical dependence after continued injection

TABLE 3.

Effects of Chemicals Related to Monoamines on Analgesic Action of AAC in Rat Tail-Flick Test. (Analgesic Test Performed 45 Minutes After Simultaneous IP of AAC and Other Compounds)

Groups	Dose (mg/kg, IP)	Change in tail-flick response (sec)
Saline + AAC	/ + 0.03	+ 1.0 ± 0.2
Pargyline‡ + AAC	75 + 0.03	+ 2.1 ± 0.6*
Selegiline + AAC	10 + 0.03	+ 0.1 ± 0.2**
Saline + saline	/ + /	0.0 ± 0.1**
Saline + AAC	/ + 0.03	+ 1.0 ± 0.0++
Apomorphine + saline	5 + /	0.0 ± 0.2+
Apomorphine + AAC	5 + 0.03	0.0 ± 0.2**
Heloperidol + saline	1 + /	0.0 ± 0.4+
Heloperidol + AAC	1 + 0.03	1.5 ± 0.3*
cAMP‡ (μg, ICV) + saline	10 + /	+ 0.2 ± 0.2+
cAMP + AAC	10 + 0.03	+ 1.6 ± 0.3*

$n = 4$-5, $\bar{x} \pm$ SD.   *$P < 0.05$,   **$P < 0.01$ versus saline + AAC group.
+$P > 0.05$,   ++$P < 0.01$ versus saline + saline group.   ‡1 hour before AAC.

of morphine (Tang et al., 1983, 1986a, 1986b). Foot-shock-induced analgesia showed a cross-tolerance to morphine-induced analgesia, but LA or DLA had no such effect (Guo & Tang, 1991). These results indicate that AAC, BUL, and LA belong to the nonnarcotic class of analgesics.

NATURAL CHOLINESTERASE INHIBITORS

Naturally occurring alkaloid galanthamine (Gal) with anti-ChE activity has been recognized in eastern European countries for nearly 40 years. In the 1960s, phytochemists of this Institute also isolated Gal and lycoramine from *Lycoris squamigera* and *L aurea* collected in eastern China. Gal has been used for many years in anesthesia and neurology (Domino, 1988; Tang & Hsu, 1966). Since ChE inhibitors as palliative agents in the treatment of Alzheimer's disease (AD) have captured the attention of many investigators (Giacobini, 1991), Gal has become the focus of extensive clinical investigation in patients with AD based on its complete oral bioavailability, long half-life, and lack of cholinergic peripheral adverse effects.

Huperzia serrata is known as the Chinese folk medicine *Qing Ceng Ta*. This herb is found chiefly in southern China, where it grows in moist places in hilly regions. The decoction of dried whole plant has been used to treat trauma, fractures, scalds, hematuria, and infections of the skin and subcutaneous tissues (Jiang Su New Medical College, 1975). Its general anesthetic activity and tran-

TABLE 4.

Anticholinesterase Activity of Natural Cholinesterase Inhibitors In Vitro.

ChEI	IC_{50} (μM)		Ratio of IC_{50}s' (BuChE/AChE)
	AChE activity	BuChE activity	
Huperzine A	0.06309	74.43	1259
Huperzine B	0.7943	125.89	158.5
N-methyl huperzine B	79.43	316.23	3.98
Galanthamine	1.995	12.59	6.3
Lycoramine	12.59	158.49	12.6
Physostigmine	0.251	1.259	5.0

AChE: rat erythrocyte membrane.   BuChE: rat serum.

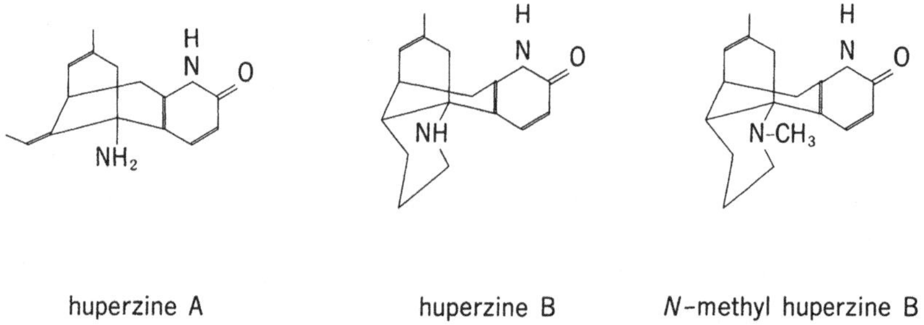

huperzine A   huperzine B   N-methyl huperzine B

Figure 2. Chemical structure of new cholinesterase inhibitors isolated from Chinese medicinal plants.

quillizing properties were found in animal experiments and in the clinic respectively. In search of the active constituent of *Huperzia serrata*, three new alkaloids, huperzine A (Hup-A), huperzine B (Hup-B), and N-methyl huperzine B(Fig. 2), with anti-ChE activities were first isolated by the Chinese (Li et al., 1987a; Liu et al., 1986). The pharmacologic effects of Hup-A and Hup-B have been studied in detail in the author's laboratory since 1982.   Hup-A and -B exhibited high selectivity toward AChE. They belong to the class of mixed and reversible ChE inhibitors (Wang et al., 1986; Xu & Tang, 1987). The inhibitory effect of Hup-A was about three and 30 times more potent than those of physostigmine and Gal with AChE, respectively.

Hup-A is the most potent AChE inhibitor as compared with other ChE inhibitors under investigation (Table 4). Hup-A can induce long-term inhibition of AChE activity and an increase in the ACh levels in brain of up to 40 % (Fig. 3). Following the administration of Hup-A, ChE activity is inhibited rather

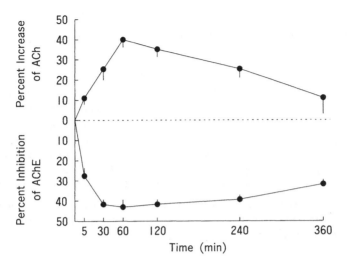

Figure 3. Time course of AChE activity and ACh levels in whole rat brain following administration of Hup-A (2 mg/kg intramuscularly). Values are expressed as percent inhibition of AChE activities or percent increase of ACh ± SEM. $n = 4$ per group.

uniformly in all brain areas, but the percent increase of ACh varies from area to area, indicating that changes in ACh levels more closely reflect the presence of cholinergic neurons and synapses than AChE activity. Hup-A did not alter the activity of choline acetyltransferase activity, indicating that the increase in levels of ACh caused by Hup-A was not likely to be mediated through an increase in the rate of synthesis of ACh (Tang et al., 1994). Hup-A at concentration of 10^{-6} to 10^{-4} does not alter the electrically evoked release of ^{3}H-ACh from cortex slices, which contrasts with the decrease of release seen with other ChE inhibitors (Tang et al., 1989). Hup-A was effective in a variety of behavioral tests designed to test an animal's learning and memory functions (Tang et al., 1988). The longest enhancing effect of Hup-A was observed in memory performance (Table 5). Hup-A-induced improvement was as potent after chronic as after acute treatment, indicating that no tolerance to the drug occurred (Fig. 4). The relative order of magnitude of the therapeutic indices of Hup-A is superior to those of physostigmine and Gal (Yan et al., 1987). Our study indicates that Hup-A more closely satisfies established criteria for an ideal ChE inhibitor for the treatment of AD than did previously tested compounds (Giacobini, 1991). On the basis of these findings, it is reasonable to consider that Hup-A is a promising candidate for clinical development as a second-generation ChE inhibitor for treating cholinergic-related neurodegenerative disorders, such as AD. The clinical trials showed

TABLE 5.

Improving Effect of ChE Inhibitor on Memory Retention of Passive Avoidance Task in Mice ($n = 10$-14)

ChEI	Dose (mg/kg)	Step-down latency (sec ± SEM)			
		24	48	72	96 (hours)
Saline	—	16.8± 2.5	19.2± 2.2	24.6± 3.2	22.5± 5.6
Huperzine A	0.2	78.8± 2.3**	34.5± 5.9*	67.1±19.9*	50.8± 8.9*
Physostigmine	0.3	66.0±13.1**	22.2± 3.7	29.0± 5.2	37.5± 7.7
Saline	—	19.4± 1.6	34.3± 4.7	21.4±19.5	37.3± 5.3
Galanthamine	2.0	48.5± 9.9**	67.8±11.8**	44.4±40.1	60.6±10.5
Tacrine	16.0	44.6± 6.1**	70.9±15.0*	31.5±33.7	59.1±14.0

*$P < 0.05$, **$P < 0.01$ versus saline. An oral dose of ChEI or saline (10ml/kg) was administered immediately after training. The retention test was performed 24, 48, 72 or 96 hours after training.

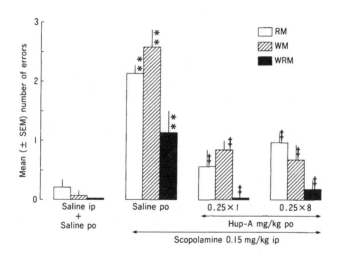

Figure 4. Effect of acute and chronic administration of Hup-A on scopolamine-induced amnesia on radial maze performance in rats ($\bar{x} \pm$ SEM). Scopolamine and Hup-A were administered 30 minutes before the test. Number of rats in bars. **$P < 0.01$ versus saline + saline. ††$P < 0.01$ versus saline + scopolamine. RM: reference memory. WM: working memory. WRM: working memory and reference memory.

a clear-cut improvement in memory following Hup-A administration in patients with age-associated memory disorders (Hanin et al.,1991). Hup-A exhibited a comparatively long duration of action and minimal side effects (Tang et al., 1994; Zhang et al., 1991). Phase II clinical trials on AD patients are in progress.

REFERENCES

Chen, W. Z., Dong, Y. L., Zhang, Y.F., Ding, G.S. (1983): Antiarrhythmic effects of Guan-Fu base A. *Acta Pharmacol. Sin.* **4**, 247-250.

Domino, E. F. (1988): Galanthamine: Another look at an old cholinesterase inhibitor. In: E. Giacobini, R. Becker (Eds.), *Current Research in Alzheimer Therapy: Cholinesterase Inhibitors*, pp. 295-303. New York: Taylor & Francis.

Giacobini, E. (1991): The second generation of cholinesterase inhibitors: Pharmacological aspects. In: R. Becker, E. Giacobini (Eds.), *Cholinergic Basis for Alzheimer Therapy*, pp. 247-262. Boston: Birkhauser.

Guo, X., Tang, X. C. (1989): Effects of central Ca^{2+} on analgesic action of lappaconitine. *Acta Pharmacol. Sin.* **10**, 504-517.

Guo, X., Tang, X. C. (1990a): Effects of reserpine and 5-HT on analgesia induced by lappaconitine and *N*-deacetyllappaconitine. *Acta Pharmacol. Sin.* **11**, 14-18.

Guo, X., Tang, X. C. (1990b): Roles of periaqueductal gray and nucleus raphe magnus on analgesia induced by lappaconitine, *N*-deacetyllappaconitine and morphine. *Acta Pharmacol. Sin.* **11**, 107-112.

Guo, X., Tang, X. C. (1991): Lappaconitine and *N*-deacetyllappaconitine potentiate footshock-induced analgesia in rats. *Life Sci.* **48**. 1365-1370.

Hanin, I., Tang, X. C., Kozikowski, A. P. (1991): Clinical and preclinical studies with huperzine. In: R. Becker, E. Giacobini (Eds.), *Cholinergic Basis for Alzheimer Therapy*, pp. 303-313. Boston: Birkhauser.

Huang, S. K., Wang, Y. E., Tang, X. C. (1983): Kinetic of neuromuscular blocking effect of dimethyl *l*-curine dimethochloride. *Acta Pharmacol. Sin.* **4**, 17-20.

Jiang Su New Medical College (1975): *Zhong Yao Da Ci Dian (Chinese Remedy Dictionary)*, pp. 215-216. Shanghai: Shanghai People's Publisher Press.

Li, J., Han, Y. Y., Liu, J. S. (1987a): Studies on the alkaloids of Qian Ceng Ta *(Huperzia Serrata)*. *Chinese Trad. Herbal Drugs*. **18**, 50-51.

Li, X. Y., Jiang, K. M., Lin, Z. Y. (1987b): Immunomodulating actions of yunaconitine. *Chinese J. Pharmacol. Toxicol.* **1**, 100-104.

Lin, Z. G., Cai, W., Tang, X. C. (1987): Antiinflammatory and analgesic actions of yunaconitine. *Chinese J. Pharmacol. Toxicol.* **1**, 93-99.

Liu, J. H., Zhu, Y. X., Tang, X. C. (1987): Anti-inflammatory and analgesic activities of *N*-deacetyllappaconitine and lappaconitine. *Acta Pharmacol. Sin.* **8**, 301-305.

Liu, J. S., Zhu, Y. L. , Yu, C. M., et al. (1986): The structure of huperzine A and B, two new alkaloids exhibiting marked anticholinesterase activity. *Can. J. Chem.* **64**, 837-839.

Lu, D. X., Guo, X., Tang, X. C. (1988): Effect of monoamine transmitters on

3-acetylaconitine analgesia. *Acta Pharmacol. Sin.* **9**, 216-220.

Shanghai Institute of Materia Medica, Academia Sinica (1979): Active principles of neuromuscular blocking actions from *Cyclea barbata, Cyclea hainanensis and Stephania epigaea* (Manispermaceae). *Ke Xue Tong Bao* **24**, 574-576.

Tang, X. C., De Sarno, P., Sugaya, K., Giacobini, E. (1989): Effect of huperzine A, a new cholinesterase inhibitor, on the central cholinergic system of the rat. *J. Neurosci. Res.* **24**, 276-285.

Tang, X. C., Feng, J., Wang, Y. E., Liu, M. Z. (1980a): Neuro-muscular blocking activity of alkaloids of *Cyclea hainanensis. Acta Pharmacol. Sin.* **1**, 17-22.

Tang, X. C., Hsu, B. (1966): The clinical application and pharmacological effect of the new drug anticholinesterase galanthamine. *Acta pharmaceut. Sin.* **13**, 68-78.

Tang, X. C., Jin, G. Z., Feng, J., et al. (1980b): Studies on the neuromuscular blocking activity of alkaloids of *Cyclea barbata* (Wall) Miers. *Acta Pharmaceut. Sin.* **9**, 513-519.

Tang, X. C., Kozikowski, A. P., Kindel, G. H., Hanin,I. (1994): Comparison of the effect of natural and synthetic huperzine A on rat brain cholinergic function *in vitro* and *in vivo. J. Ethnopharmacol.* **44**, 147-155.

Tang, X. C., Lin, Z. G., Cai, W., et al. (1984): Antiinflammatory effect of 3-acetylaconitine. *Acta Pharmacol. Sin.* **5**. 85-89.

Tang, X. C., Liu, X. J., Feng, J., et al. (1986a): Analgesic action and no physical dependenece of 3-acetylacontine. *Acta Pharmacol. Sin.* **7**, 413-418.

Tang, X. C., Liu, X. J., Lu, W. H., et al. (1986b): Studies on the analgesic action and physical dependence of bullyaconitine A. *Acta Pharmaceut. Sin.* **21**, 886-891.

Tang, X. C., Xiong, Z. Q., Qian, B. C., et al. (1994): Cognition improvement by oral huperzine A: A novel acetylcholinesterase inhibitor. In: E. Giacobini, R. Becker (Eds.), *Alzheimer Therapy: Therapeutic Strategies*, pp. 113-119. Boston: Birkhauser.

Tang, X. C., Zhu, M.Y., Feng, J. (1983): Studies on the pharmacological action of lappaconitine hydrobromide. *Acta Pharmaceut. Sin.* **18**, 579-584.

Tang. X. C., Zhu, X. D., Lu, W. H. (1988): Studies on the nootropic effects of huperzine A and B: Two selective AChE inhibitors. In: E. Giacobini, R. Becker (Eds.), *Current Research in Alzheimer Therapy: Cholinesterase Inhibitors*, pp. 289-293. New York: Taylor & Francis.

Tang, Z. J., Lao, A. N., Chen, Y., et al. (1980c): Studies on the active principle of neuromuscular blocking actions of *Cyclea barbata* (Wall) Miers. *Acta Pharmaceut. Sin.* **15**. 506-508.

Wang, F. P. (1981a): A review of the chemical studies on the alkaloids from *Aconitum* and *Delphinium* plants. *Acta Pharmaceut. Sin.* **16**. 943-959.

Wang, J. W. (1981b): Clinical trials on the muscular relaxant dimethyl-*l*-curine-dimethochloride (412 cases). *Chinese Trad. Herbal Drugs* **12**, 26-30.

Wang, Y. E., Yue, D. X., Tang, X. C. (1986): Anticholinesterase activity of huperzine A. *Acta Pharmacol. Sin.* **7**, 110-113.

Xu, H., Tang, X. C. (1987): Anticholinesterase activity of huperzine B. *Acta Pharmacol. Sin.* **8**. 18-22.

Yan, X. F., Lu, W. H., Luo, W. J., Tang, X. C. (1987): Effect of huperzine A and

B on skeletal muscle and electroencephalography. *Acta Pharmacol. Sin.* **8,** 117-123.

Yang, Q. Z., Lin, L. R. (1981): Mode of action of dimethy-*l*-curine dimethochloride on neuromuscular transmission. *Acta Pharmacol. Sin.* **2,** 19-23.

Zhang, R. W., Tang, X. C., Han, Y. Y., et al. (1991): Drug evaluation of huperaine A in the treatment of senile memory disorders. *Acta Pharmacol. Sin.* **12,** 250-252.

4

A Double-Blind Control Study of Huperzine A and Piracetam in Patients with Age-Associated Memory Impairment and Dementias

Zuxin Wang, Guiying Ren, Youwen Zhao, Yaqin Weng, Mingchen Ding, Xinqing Zhang, Chen Meng, Peijie Yang, Zhongxuan Wu, Jianping Wang, Baozhu Li, Yunru Zhang, Ruicheng Hua, Jianan Wei, Shuzhen Huang, Shuhua Fei, Baorong Fan, Shulan Wang, Xiangping Ma, and Qian Xia

Huperzine A tablet is a reversible potent acetylcholinesterase (AChE) inhibitor developed by the Institute of Toxicology and Pharmaceutics, Academy of Military Medical Science, Chinese People's Liberation Army. This was a clinical trial of huperzine A carried out by the Institute of Mental Health, Beijing Medical University; Xuan Wu Hospital, Capital Medical College; Guang An Men Hospital, Academy of Traditional Chinese Medicine; Beijing An Ding Hospital; and Beijing Friendship Hospital from October 1990 to August 1992. The purpose of the study was to compare huperzine's efficacy and safety in patients with memory disorders of middle and old age, as well as various demented patients, by using piracetam as a control.

There were 131 patients in the huperzine A group (group A), including 67 patients with benign memory disorder and 64 patients with organic dementia. Of the 81 patients in the Piracetam group (group B), 34 had benign memory disorder and 47 organic dementia.

The improvement rate and significant improvement rate for benign memory disorder were 83.6% and 73.2% respectively.

For organic dementia, the memory improvement rate and marked improvement rate were 62.5% and 53.1%. Improvement and marked improvement for cognitive function were 31.3% and 25.0%. Dizziness, nausea, and gastrointestinal symptoms are the major side effects of huperzine A. The incidence of side effects as a whole is 4.7 - 7.7% ; no significant differences were seen as compared with Piracetam. The study shows that huperzine A is an effective and safe drug for memory disorders in both middle-aged and elderly persons and in patients with dementia.

METHODS

This was a multicenter collaborative study with a unified design. Investigators involved in the study were trained prior to the study and the scales used were agreed upon. The coefficient of correlation was 0.87 ($P < 0.05$).

1. Inclusion criteria:
   A. Patients were male or female with memory and intelligence disorders. Benign memory disorder group: The only complaint was forgetfulness, among those over 50 years old. Organic demented group: Including cerebral vascular dementia; Alzheimer's disease (AD) and other dementias that meet the *Chinese Classification and Diagnostic Criteria of Mental Disorders*, second edition (CCMD-2) (Yang, 1989).
   B. No severe heart, hepatic, or renal dysfunction.
   C. Memory quotient (MQ) ≤ 90.

2. Medications:
   Huperzine A tablets (each tablet contains 50 μg huperzine A) provided by the Institute of Toxicology and Pharmaceutics, Academy of Military Medical Science, Chinese People's Liberation Army. Coded as No. 1. Piracetam capsule, produced by Red Star Pharmaceutic Company, Chang Chun City. Each capsule contains 0.2 g. Coded as No. 2.

3. Procedures:
   A. Benign memory disorder group: Patients were randomly divided into two subgroups after all required tests and examinations were completed. Huperzine A group (group A): Huperzine A tablets were given, 100-150 μg, two to three times a day for four weeks. The daily mean dose was about 300 μg. Piracetam group (group B): Capsules, 1.6-3.2 g/day divided into two to three doses, were given. The daily mean dose was 2.4 g.
   B. Organic dementia group: Also randomly divided into two subgroups. No nootropics or drugs that affect cerebral metabolism and functioning were taken except Huperzine A: 100-150 μg, two to three times a day for six weeks. Piracetam: 1.6-3.2 g/day for six weeks.

4. Method:
   A. Examinations before the study:
      (1) History collection, physical and neurologic examinations.
      (2) Laboratory tests, including hemoglobin (Hb), white blood count

(WBC), hepatic and renal functions, electrocardiogram (ECG), electroencephalogram (EEG) or computed tomography (CT) scan.

(3) Psychological tests with structured rating scales, such as clinical memory scale (Xu, 1984) and Mini-Mental State Examination (MMSE). The MMSE was used for dementias only.

B. Examinations at the end of study: All the examinations and tests mentioned above were repeated.

C. Side effects were evaluated at the end of the first, third and last week of the study.

D. Efficacy evaluation: Made by physicians in charge at the end of study. The evaluation criteria were as follows:

(1) Efficacy of memory improvement: The MQ increased rate combined with clinical impression was used to evaluate the efficacy of memory improvement.

$$\text{MQ increased rate} = \frac{\text{MQ after treatment} - \text{MQ before treatment}}{\text{MQ before treatment}} \times 100\%$$

Improved: Clinically improved and the rate of MQ increased $\geq 12\%$.
Markedly improved: Much greater clinical improvement and the rate of MQ increased $\geq 20\%$.
Not improved: No change clinically and the rate of MQ score increased $< 12\%$.

(2) Efficacy of cognitive functioning was evaluated with both clinical impression and MMSE.

$$\text{MMSE increased rate} = \frac{\text{MMSE score after treatment} - \text{score before treatment}}{\text{MMSE score before treatment}} \times 100\%$$

Improved: Clinically improved and the rate of MMSE score increased $\geq 12\%$.
Markedly improved: Much greater clinical improvement and the rate of MMSE score increased $\geq 20\%$.
Not improved: No change clinically and the rate of MMSE score increased $< 12\%$.

E. Data analysis: All the data collected were statistically analyzed with ANALYST package and χ^2 and t-tests were carried out to determine the significance of difference.

RESULTS

1. General data:

A. 131 patients in group A and 81 patients in group B. There were no significant differences between the groups.

B. No singnificant difference with regard to gender, age, education, and course of illness were found between the A and B groups (Table 1, Table 2).

2. Clinical assessment result for benign memory disorder:

A. Efficacy regarding memory improvement:

There were 67 patients in group A. The total improvement rate was 83.6% and the marked improvement rate was 73.2% with 16.4% not improved. Both total improvement and marked improvement rates were significantly higher than for group B (Table 3).

B. Results on the clinical memory scale assessment:

After treatment with huperzine A, scores on all subitems of the clinical memory scale, the total score, and the MQ score were significantly higher than before treatment in group A. The scores on directed memory, picture recall, nonsensical pattern recognition, total score, and MQ were significantly higher than in group B (Table 4).

C. MQ rank assessment results:

The number of patients in the higher score rank in group A was much greater after treatment than before. No MQ was in the normal range before treatment; after treatment, the percentage of MQ in the normal range increased to 70.2%. There was a significant difference as compared with group B (Table 5).

D. Correlation analysis of efficacy with both MQ increased rate and MQ rank:

There are highly positive correlations of efficacy with both the MQ increased rate and MQ rank for groups A and B (Table 6).

3. Clinical assessment result of patients with organic dementia

A. Analysis of efficacy on memory:

(1) Clinical analysis: At the end of the study, the total improvement rate and significant improvement rate for group A was 62.5% and 53.1%, respectively, higher than for group B. However, there was no significant difference (Table 7).

(2) Clinical memory scale assessment: The total score, score on all subitems of the scale (except portrait recall), and MQ were much higher after treatment than before in group A. No significant differences were found between group A and group B (Table 8, Table 9).

(3) MQ rank assessment: No MQ in group A, was in the normal range before treatment; after treatment, the percentage increased to 21.1%. However, no significant difference was found as compared with group B (Table 10).

(4) Correlation analysis of memory improvement with MQ increased rate and MQ rank: There were highly positive correlations among memory efficacy, MQ increased rate, and MQ rank for both groups (Table 11).

B. Efficacy of cognitive function

(1) Clinical analysis: The total improvement rate and significant improvement rate for group A were 31.3% and 25.0% respectively. There was no significant difference in terms of significant improvement rate as compared with group B (Table 12).

(2) MMSE assessment: The score on the MMSE for group A was slightly higher after treatment than before treatment, with no significant difference between them in either group A or B (Table 13, Table 14).

(3) Correlation analysis of efficacy on cognitive function and increased MMSE score: There were significant correlations of efficacy on cognitive function and increased MMSE scores in both groups (Table 15)

C. Side effects

The side effects of huperzine A and piracetam were measured at the first, third, and last week of treatment. The main side effects of huperzine A are dizziness (0.8-3.1%), and gastrointestinal symptoms (2.3-3.1%). Side effects of all types combined are 4.7-7.7%. There is no significant difference as compared with piracetam (Table 16).

D. Laboratory tests

There was no significant change in the Hb, WBC, hepatic and renal functions, ECG and EEG at the end of the study, as compared with before treatment, for patients in group A.

DISCUSSION

Huperzine A, a new alkaloid extracted from *Huperzia serrata*, is a revessible potent AChE inhibitor exhibits selective inhibition on AChE. The inhibitory effect is three times greater than for physostigmine and 30 times greater than for galanthamine in rats with relative low toxicity (Wang et al., 1986). Experimentally, it induced EEG activation, facilitating the learning and retrieval process of discrimination performance (Tang et al., 1986; Lu et al., 1988). A clinical trial carried out by Zhang of aged patients with memory impairment demonstrated that huperzine A, 30 μg injection, had definite memory-enhancing effects, better than hydergine 600 μg (Zhang, 1986). Our study showed huperzine A tablets produced similar results. The total improvement rate for age-associated memory impairment or benign memory disorder was 83.6%; total scores on both the Clinical Memory Scale and MQ increased significantly after a four-week treatment, with a significant difference as compared with piracetam.

For dementia as a whole, the memory improvement rate on the Clinical Memory Scale was 62.5% and 53.1% respectively. However, the improvement and marked improvement rates for huperzine A for cognitive function as measured by the MMSE was only 31.3% and 25.0%; no significant differences exist as compared with piracetam.

MID and AD are the major category of dementia. Our study appeared to show that the effect of huperzine A on MID is somewhat better than on AD in terms of both memory and cognitive function. AD is defined as a degenerative organic mental disease with diffuse brain deterioration and dementia. Although the cause of AD has not yet been clarified, many of its symptoms have been related to neurotransmitter changes, particularly in the cholinergic system (Perry, 1988). Huperzine A as a potent AChE inhibitor might be of some advantage for AD. Therefore, a three month-longer treatment course, a higher dosage range, and a larger sample size, as well as a number of international standardized cognitive function assessment instruments, should be utilized for further studies.

REFERENCES

Lu, W., Shou, J., Tang, X. (1988): Improving effect of huperzine A on discrimination performance in aged rats with experimental cognitive impairment. *Acta Pharmacol. Sin.*, **9** (1), 11-15.

Perry, E. K. (1986): The cholinergic hypothesis—10 years on. *Br. Med. Bull.* **42,** 63-69.

Tang, X., Han, Y., Chen, X., Zhu, X. (1986): Effects of huperzine A on learning and retrieval process of discrimination performance in rats. *Acta Pharmacol. Sin.*, **17**, 507-511.

Wang, Y., Yue, D., Tang, X. (1986): Anticholinesterase activity. *Acta Pharmacol. Sin.*, **7** (2), 110-113.

Xu, S. (1984): *Clinical Memory Scale Manual*. Institute of Psychology. Chinese Academy of Science., Shanghai.

Yang, D. (1989): *Chinese Classification and Diagnostic Criteria of Mental Disorders* (2 nd ed). Hunan University Press.

Zhang, S. (1986): Therapeutic effects of huperzine A on the aged with memory impairment. *New Drugs Clini. Reme.* **5** (5), 260-262.

TABLE 1.

Comparison of Patients in Groups A and B

	Group A		Group B		x^2	P
	N	%	N	%		
Benign memory disorder	67	51.1	34	42.1		
Organic dementia						
Multi-infarct dementia (MID)	36	27.5	35	43.2		
AD	18	13.7	4	4.9		
Others	10	7.7	8	9.8		
Total	64	48.9	47	57.9		
Total	131		81		1.69	0.20

TABLE 2.

Comparison of Groups as to Gender, Age, Education and Course of Illness

	Group A (n=131)		Group B (n=81)		χ^2	P
	N	%	N	%		
Gender						
Male	95	72.5	53	65.4		
Female	36	27.5	28	34.6		
Total	131	100	81	100	0.88	0.35
Education						
Illiterate	13	9.9	13	16.1		
Primary school	37	28.2	30	37.0		
High school	50	38.2	27	33.3		
College	31	23.7	11	13.6		
Total	131	100	81	100	5.65	0.13
Course (year)						
0.5-1	33	25.2	16	19.8		
1-2	31	23.6	30	37.0		
2-3	20	15.3	14	17.3		
>3	47	35.9	21	25.9		
Total	131	100	81	100	5.42	0.14
Mean age						
Benign memory disorder	63.6±6.4		65.9±6.1			0.11
	(50-79 years old)		(52-76 years old)			
Organic dementia	62.9±6.8		62.4±6.3			0.68
	(50-80 years old)		(50-76 years old)			

TABLE 3.

Improvement in Memory for Patients with Benign Memory Disorder

	Group A (n=67)		Group B (n=34)		χ^2	P
	N	%	N	%		
Total improvement	56	83.6	17	50.0	12.69	0.001
Marked improvement	49	73.5	11	32.4	15.55	0.001
No improvement	11	16.4	17	50.0		

TABLE 4.

Clinical Memory Scale Assessment for Patients with Benign Memory Disorder

	Group A ($n=67$)			Group B ($n=34$)		
	Before treatment	After treatment	Score increased	Before treatment	After treatment	Score increased
Directed memory	10.1± 4.6	18.0± 5.1	7.9± 5.3[ac]	10.6± 4.7	13.5± 5.9	2.9± 5.4[b]
Associated learning	11.9± 3.9	16.5± 3.7	4.6± 3.7[a]	11.3± 3.7	15.4± 4.9	4.1± 4.8[b]
Picture recall	12.4± 5.3	16.4± 5.9	4.0± 3.7[ac]	12.4± 5.6	12.5± 4.6	0.1± 5.9
Nonsensical-pattern recognition	14.0± 6.3	19.3± 6.1	5.3± 6.8[ac]	16.3± 6.3	16.4± 6.0	0.1± 6.0
Portrait recall	11.9± 6.4	14.9± 4.4	3.0± 6.7[a]	11.8± 5.9	12.4± 7.0	0.6± 7.4
Total score	60.9±14.6	85.8±16.6	24.9±13.8[ac]	62.4±13.6	69.7±19.5	7.3±15.0
MQ	76.3±12.1	97.7±15.3	21.4±11.6[ac]	79.0± 9.7	85.9±14.2	6.9±13.6[b]
MQ increased			29.8±20.7[c]			9.7±18.3

[a] After treatment with hyperzine A, the score was significantly higher than before.

[b] After treatment with piracetam, the score was significantly higher than before.

[c] The score increased for group A significantly more than for group B

TABLE 5.

Distribution of Patients Based on MQ Rank for Benign Memory Disorder

	Group A ($n=67$)				Group B ($n=34$)			
MQ rank	Before treatment		After treatment		Before treatment		After treatment	
	N	%	N	%	N	%	N	%
Very poor (≤69)	14	20.9	2	3.0	6	17.6	6	17.6
Poor (70-79)	21	31.3	9	13.4	10	29.4	4	11.7
Below the middle (80-90)	32	47.8	9	13.4	18	53.0	12	35.3
Total	67	100.0	20	29.8	34	100.0	22	64.6
Normal (91-109)	0		33	49.3	0		10	29.4
Above the middle (110-119)	0		13	19.4	0		2	6.0
Excellent (≥120)	0		1	1.5	0		0	
Total	0		47	70.2	0		12	35.4

Comparison of group A patients before and after treatment: $P < 0.01$ ($\mu = 8.95$).

Comparison of group B patients before and after treatment: $P < 0.01$ ($\mu = 4.32$).

Comparison of group A and group B after treatment: $P < 0.01$ ($\mu = 3.51$).

TABLE 6.

Correlation Analysis of Efficacy for Patients with Benign Memory Disorder

	Group A	Group B
Efficacy compared with MQ increased rate	0.83*	0.86*
Efficacy compared with MQ rank	0.70*	0.57*

$*P<0.001$

TABLE 7.

Clinical Analysis of Memory Improvement for Patients with Organic Dementia

	Group A ($n=64$)		Group B ($n=47$)		χ^2	P
	N	%	N	%		
Total improved	40	62.5	25	53.2	0.88	0.50
Significantly improved	34	53.1	20	42.6	0.13	0.70
Unchanged	24	37.5	22	46.8		

TABLE 8.

Clinical Memory Scale Assessment of Organic Dementia

	Group A ($n=64$)			Group B ($n=47$)		
	Before treatment	After treatment	Score increased	Before treatment	After treatment	Score increased
Directed memory	8.0± 4.0	12.3± 6.8	4.3± 5.5[a]	10.5± 5.4	14.0± 5.7	3.5± 4.1[b]
Associated learning	8.9± 5.2	11.9± 6.4	3.0± 4.8[a]	10.8± 6.2	14.1± 6.3	3.2± 4.1[b]
Picture recall	6.9± 6.0	9.7± 7.4	2.9± 4.4[a]	9.8± 5.5	11.4± 5.9	1.6± 5.8
Nonsensical-figure recognition	10.8± 7.0	13.3± 7.7	2.5± 7.8[a]	14.5± 7.6	15.4± 7.8	0.9±10.1
Portrait recall	9.4± 7.3	10.4± 6.4	1.0± 7.0	10.7± 6.6	10.5± 7.8	−0.2±7.5
Total score	43.6±20.6	58.6±28.9	15.0±16.3[a]	56.3±19.6	65.4±24.0	9.1±19.9[b]
MQ	61.4±16.1	74.0±22.8	12.6±13.5[a]	69.7±16.1	77.9±19.7	8.3±16.5[b]
Increased MQ rate			20.6±22.7		14.1±26.4	14.1±26.4

[a] Score after treatment significantly higher than before treatment for group A ($P<0.05$).

[b] Score after treatment significantly higher than before treatment for group B ($P<0.05$).

TABLE 9.

Comparison of MQ Increased Rate Between Group A and Group B

	Group A	Group B
Benign memory disorder	29.8 ± 20.7[a]	9.7 ± 18.3
MID	23.7 ± 20.3[a]	13.9 ± 24.4
AD	16.9 ± 21.7	14.3 ± 34.4
Other dementia	23.7 ± 20.3	13.9 ± 24.4

[a] MQ increased rate in group A significantly higher than in group B

TABLE 10.

Distribution of Patients Based on MQ Rank for Organic Dementias

MQ rank	Group A ($n=64$)				Group B ($n=47$)			
	Before treatment		After treatment		Before treatment		After treatment	
	N	%	N	%	N	%	N	%
Very poor (≤ 69)	39	60.9	28	43.8	19	40.4	16	34.0
Poor (70-79)	16	25.0	10	15.6	13	27.7	8	17.0
Below the middle (80-90)	9	14.1	8	12.5	15	31.9	12	25.6
Total	64	100.0	46	71.9	47	100.0	36	76.6
Normal (91-109)	0		13	20.3	0		8	17.0
Above the middle (110-119)	0		5	7.8	0		2	4.3
Excellent (≥ 120)	0		0		0		1	2.1
Total	0		18	28.1	0		11	23.4

Comparison of Group A patients before and after treatment: $P < 0.01 (\mu = 5.0)$.
Comparison of Group B patients before and after treatment: $P < 0.01 (\mu = 3.79)$.
Comparison of group A and group B: $P > 0.05 (\mu = 0.56)$.

TABLE 11.

Correlation of Efficacy with MQ Increased Rate and MQ Rank in Organic Dementia

	Group A	Group B
Efficacy and increased MQ rate	0.84*	0.80*
Efficacy and MQ rank	0.43*	0.50*

* $P < 0.001$

TABLE 12.

Cognitive Function Improvement in Organic Dementia

	Group A ($n=64$)		Group B ($n=47$)		χ^2	P
	N	%	N	%		
Total improved	20	31.3	24	51.0	4.44	0.03
Significantly improved	16	25.0	12	25.5	0.01	0.85
Unchanged	44	68.7	23	49.0		

TABLE 13.

MMSE Assessment of Organic Dementia

	Group A ($n=64$)	Group B ($n=47$)
Before treatment	19.7 ± 6.8	21.4 ± 6.9
After treatment	20.7 ± 6.9	22.2 ± 6.9
Score increased	1.0 ± 3.7	1.0 ± 3.1

TABLE 14.

Comparison of MMSE Score Change in Group A and Group B Before and After Treatment

	Group A ($n=64$)			Group B ($n=47$)		
	Before treatment	After treatment	Score increased	Before treatment	After treatment	Score increased
MID	20.6 ± 6.2	22.5 ± 5.9	1.9 ± 3.8	22.6 ± 6.0	23.7 ± 5.9	1.5 ± 2.4
AD	16.1 ± 6.3	15.8 ± 5.9	-0.3 ± 6.1	12.0 ± 5.0	13.8 ± 5.3	1.8 ± 1.3
Others	25.1 ± 5.5	26.4 ± 5.0	1.3 ± 3.1	24.8 ± 4.4	24.3 ± 6.2	-0.5 ± 4.9

TABLE 15.

Correlation of Efficacy and Cognitive Functions of Patients with Organic Dementia

	Group A	Group B
Efficacy and increased MMSE score	0.78*	0.68*

* $P < 0.001$

TABLE 16.
Comparison of Side Effects of Huperzine A and Piracetam

First week						
	Group A		Group B		χ^2	P
	N	%	N	%		
None	121	92.2	76	93.9	0.16	0.69
Gastrointestinal symptoms	4	3.1	0		2.52	0.11
Dizziness	3	2.3	4	4.9	1.09	0.30
Headache	1	0.8	0	0	0.62	0.43
Distress, thoracic	1	0.8	1	1.2	0.12	0.73
Dry mouth, insomnia	1	0.8	0		0.62	0.43
Fatigue	0		0			

Third week						
	Group A		Group B		χ^2	P
	N	%	N	%		
None	122	93.0	79	97.6	1.91	0.15
Gastrointestinal symptoms	3	2.3	0		1.88	0.17
Dizziness	3	2.3	1	1.2	0.71	0.40
Headache	1	0.8	0		0.62	0.43
Distress, thoracic	0		1	1.2	1.62	0.20
Dry mouth, insomnia	0		0			
Fatigue	1	0.8	0		0.62	0.43
Gastrointestinal symptom and thoracic distress	1	0.8	0		0.62	0.43

Last week						
	Group A		Group B		χ^2	P
	N	%	N	%		
None	125	95.3	78	96.3	0.09	0.91
Gastrointestinal symptoms	3	2.3	0		1.88	0.17
Dizziness	1	0.8	2	2.5	1.04	0.31
Headache	0		0			
Distress, thoracic	1	0.8	1	1.2	0.12	0.73
Gastrointestinal symptoms and thoracic distress	1	0.8	0		0.62	0.43
Dry mouth, insomnia	0		0			
Fatigue	0		0			

5

Medicinal Plants: A Potential Source of New Psychotherapeutic Drugs*

Jerry Cott and Renuka Misra

An appreciation of the history of psychopharmacology involves recognition of naturally occurring compounds, particularly medicinal plants. In 1990, the National Institute of Mental Health (NIMH) established a contract to facilitate the pharmacologic profiling of potential new synthetic drugs and natural product extracts. This screening contract provides state-of-the-art in vitro assays for up to 100 different central nervous system (CNS) receptors. Because of the prohibitive cost of random screening, it was determined that natural products research should be based on the availability of ethnopharmacologic information. Natural product extracts would be selected for initial receptor screening based on their traditional or folkloric use for various mental disorders. In addition to empirical human data suggesting their efficacy in a psychiatric disorder, the number of potential drug candidates could then be narrowed down by applying various selection constraints; for example, there should be evidence of pharmacologic activity consistent with the purported therapeutic effect and either a history of safe human use or animal toxicology data on which to base an approximate risk-benefit ratio.

Although the initial results are encouraging, more studies are necessary to determine the relation between these binding data and the reported pharmacologic effects. Analyses of the individual compounds or groups of compounds are also needed for most medicinal plants to determine whether their safety and efficacy can be increased. In examples where the whole plant or crude extract is superior (such as with Ginkgo biloba*), the Food and Drug Admin-*

* Presented at the Symposium on New Drug Development from Herbal Medicines in Neuropsychopharmacology of the 19th CINP Congress, June 27–July 1, 1994, Washington D.C.

istration (FDA) regulatory requirements pose additional barriers to development, since proof of the safety and efficacy of each individual chemical, as well as of the combination(s) of those chemicals, would be necessary in order to demonstrate synergy. The inability to obtain patent exclusivity for plants that have been reported in the literature results in disinterest by the major pharmaceutical companies. These difficulties are yet to be overcome in the United States. Among traditional medical practitioners in such countries as China, it is generally accepted that acute illnesses may be best treated with Western medicine, while chronic disorders should be treated with less toxic, traditional treatments which are generally aimed at correcting the presumed underlying cause. Although Westerners do not commonly categorize illnesses in this manner, there is a persuasive logic to this dichotomy. Demonstration of efficacy in chronic disorders, however, will probably be more difficult, owing to the need for longer trials, more naturalistic indices of health and quality of life, and outcome measures that go beyond the relief of symptoms. Such countries as Germany, France, and Japan have developed approval processes specifically for phytomedicinals. Moreover, the World Health Organization (WHO) has released Guidelines for the Assessment of Herbal Medicines. The United States should consider the adoption of a similar registration process to encourage new drug development in this country.

INTRODUCTION

Despite the advances made in the past three decades in utilizing synthetic chemical approaches to drug design and sophisticated structure-activity studies, there is still a great need in the field of medicine for novel compounds with unique mechanisms of action. While many thousands of structural analogs have been synthesized and tested, numerous gaps remain in the therapeutic armamentarium for psychiatric illnesses. The majority of new drugs marketed for psychotherapeutic indications in recent years have been only incremental improvements on existing medications. Major breakthroughs have resulted primarily from the study of natural products, as well as serendipity. Some of our most valuable drugs have been isolated from plant and animal sources. These include aspirin, morphine, reserpine (the first antipsychotic), almost all of our antibiotics, digitalis, and a number of anticancer agents, including vincristine, vinblastine, and taxol. In North America, a quarter of all prescriptions written are for plant products or for products based on plants, and 75% of these are used in ways that directly correlate with their traditional uses by native cultures; that is, they were "discovered" by investigating folklore claims (Farnsworth et al., 1985).

Why has interest in natural products research as a method of drug discovery declined? In the early 1900s, pharmaceutical firms and academic investigators were engaged in the collection and testing of natural products for biologic activity. In the 18th century, Benjamin Rush, the father of American psychiatry and personal physician to George Washington, carried out extensive investigations of medicines used by the Native Americans (Rush, 1774). With the exception of drug treatments for cancer and the acquired immune deficiency syndrome (AIDS), natural product investigations have been largely curtailed in recent years. There are many reasons for the decline in research. The primary reason is financial; herbs cannot be patented, and drug companies thus are not motivated to invest money in their testing and promotion. Random screening of biologic materials in the search for potentially patentable compounds (those not previously described in the medical literature) is very expensive and has a low rate of return. Another reason may be more philosophic, and may be due to the way in which medicine is currently perceived and taught in American medical schools. Former Surgeon General C. Everett Koop stated, "Medicine today has its problems and its high-tech achievements because of the Flexner Report of 1910."[1] That document criticized American medical schools for lax standards and resulted in great changes in the ways in which medicine and science were taught. This conservative scientific approach was not consistent with the use of anecdotal information or case histories in the development of new treatment modalities. Soft data of this type have been almost totally replaced by biochemical assays and preclinical animal studies, followed by placebo-controlled clinical trials for the determination of therapeutic activity. Unfortunately, we lose a great deal of valuable information when these anecdotal human data are overlooked. As Eugene Garfield proposed in a recent commentary,[2] anecdotal evidence has provided a major function in subsequent "breakthrough advances benefiting public health." In contrast, Germany currently requires all physicians to pass a section on herbal medicine before becoming licensed (Blumenthal, 1992).

The principal role played by anecdote and serendipity is more apparent in the early history of psychopharmacology than in any other field of medicine. Examples include the antipsychotic effects of chlorpromazine (originally developed as an adjunct to anesthesia) (Lehmann & Hanrahan, 1954) and the antidepressant activity of imipramine (Kuhn, 1958) (both developed originally for their sedative, antihistamine properties); the unexpected antidepressant activity of iproniazid (originally developed for the treatment of tuberculosis and later found

---

[1]"We need to teach doctors to care." In *The Washington Post Parade Magazine*, July 3, 1994.

[2]"Case histories: A valuable testament to the importance of biomedical research." In *The Scientist*, July 11. 1994.

to inhibit monoamine oxidase [MAO]) (Selikoff et al., 1952; Loomer et al., 1957); and the antimanic effects of lithium (discovered during attempts to solubilize urates in guinea pigs) (Cade, 1949).

An appreciation of the history of pharmacology also involves an appreciation of naturally occurring compounds, primarily in medicinal plants. Pharmacology itself began with attempts to understand the valuable biologic properties of medicinal plants. Natural products research is dependent on other disciplines, such as medicinal chemistry, ethnobotany (the study of the relationship between humans and their ambient vegetation), and ethnopharmacology (the study of the use of plants and animals for their toxic or medicinal properties by local cultures and peoples). The "discovery" of psychoactive products—such as curare, atropine, ouabain, morphine, reserpine, and digitalis—and their introduction into modern medicine were really a rediscovery. Although Western medicine in general did not adopt these drugs until this century, many of them are ancient medicinals. The use of *Rauwolfia serpentina* dates back almost 3000 years to ancient Hindu Ayurvedic medicine as a treatment for insanity and other disorders. The first scientific description of reserpine as a tranquilizer was given in 1931 (Sen & Bose, 1931). The alkaloid was first isolated from root extracts of *R serpentina* in 1952 (Müller et al., 1952) and its structure described in 1954 (Dorfman et al., 1954), Nathan Kline pioneered its use in the Western world in 1954 (Kline, 1954). for which he won the prestigious Albert Lasker Prize in 1957. Pursuit of the mechanism of action of reserpine led Arvid Carlsson, at the University of Göteborg, Sweden, to the discovery of a new CNS transmitter, dopamine (Carlsson, 1959). Carlsson provided evidence that dopamine, previously believed to be only a precursor in the synthesis of norepinephrine, not only was a transmitter, but that its insufficiency resulted in the mysterious neurologic disturbances of Parkinson's disease. Carlsson's investigations into the mechanism of the antipsychotic activities of reserpine and chlorpromazine led him to propose that the "neuroleptic" mechanism was a blockade of brain dopamine receptors (Carlsson & Lindqvist, 1963). Thus, the overactivity of dopamine systems might be associated with schizophrenia. Carlsson won the 1994 Japan Prize (the Japanese equivalent of the Nobel prize) for his pioneering work.

Together with serendipity, psychoactive medicinal plants have provided opportunities for discoveries in neuroscience, including new neurotransmitters and receptors, second messengers, and ion channels. A significant scientific constraint is placed on drug development when we must limit our search to synthetic chemicals that interact with known biologic systems in predicable ways. Truly unique medications are unlikely to emerge. This is especially true of research in areas where there are no effective drug treatments, such as cognitive disorders. This lack impedes even the incremental "me too" advances associated with the purely synthetic approoch.

Recent global economic and environmental pressures are also the cause of a renewed interest in natural products research. Perhaps the most compelling of these is the rapid disappearance of the flora and fauna of the tropical rain forests; if these natural sources of phytomedicinals are not explored now, they may disappear forever. The tropical rain forests contain the most diverse collection of plants in the world; as much as 16% of the total plant species on the planet may be contained in the five million square kilometers of tropical America (Soejarto & Farnsworth, 1989). It is noteworthy that the U.S. Congress demonstrated its interest in unconventional medical practices by establishing the National Institutes of Health (NIH) Office of Alternative Medicine. In his survey of the prevalence of unconventional medicine treatments sought by the American public, David Eisenberg demonstrated that these holistic practices can no longer be ignored (Eisenberg et al., 1993).

The herbal products industry racked up over $1 billion in retail sales in the United States,[3] where consumers also paid more than $8 billion in 1980 for prescriptions containing active principles obtained from plants (Farnsworth et al., 1985). While a few herbs and isolated compounds are approved for use as over-the-counter (OTC) drug ingredients, most herbal products are regulated and sold as foods. According to the FDA, any product that is used for the prevention, treatment, mitigation, or cure of any disease condition is considered a drug. Drug approval costs in the United States are extremely high. Since botanicals are not patentable, and are very complex chemically, neither pharmaceutical companies nor herb companies, which lack the financial resources to overcome the regulatory obstacles, consider them viable candidates for drug approval.

No complex natural product has been approved as a new drug since the 1962 Kefauver-Harris amendments were enacted. European and Asian countries have introduced hundreds of botanical remedies in this time, some of which are among the most widely used medicines in their health care systems (McCaleb, 1994),

NATURAL PRODUCTS RESEARCH AT NIMH

The 1988 National Advisory Mental Health Council (NAMHC) Report to Congress on the Decade of the Brain[4] provides the background for the current interest and activities in natural products research. The NAMHC recommended that NIMH cooperate with the National Cancer Institute (NCI) to obtain representative samples that are being collected under their natural products collection program and to formulate specific plans for a natural products screening program to be implemented through a series of contracts.

---

[3]Industry survey, American Herbal Products Association, 1991.

[4]"Approaching the 21st Century: Opportunities for NIMH Neuroscience Research." DHHS Publication No. (ADM) 88-1580 (1988).

In response to the NIMH Council, the Psychotherapeutic Drug Discovery & Development Program was established in 1991. Since no money was set aside for these initiatives, a program announcement[5] mentioning natural products research, released in the same year, had to compete for available research funds within the Institute. Other ways of providing support were sought. An example of this was the joint (NIH, USAID, National Science Foundation) Request for Applications concerning biodiversity preservation, natural products research, and economic development released in 1993.[6]

A workshop entitled "The Potential for Deriving New Psychotherapeutic Medications from Natural Products" was sponsored by the NIMH in April 1992. This workshop assembled many notable natural product scientists from academia and from the other Institutes of the NIH to assist in the planning of this initiative and to determine how to achieve its goals while staying within its limited financial resources. Representatives from the large natural products program of the NCI shared their experience and agreed to make their library of plant samples available to the NIMH. The NCI approach to natural products research was presented as a random, large-scale screening of biologic samples through specific tumor cell cultures. Unfortunately, predictive, high-capacity assays are not available for mental illnesses. They are sometimes even questionable for anticancer agents. One of the slides presented by NCI read:

> "We may not be able to cure human cancers, but if there is ever an epidemic of L1210 Leukemia in mice, the cures are waiting."
> *—Anonymous NCI staffer*

Thus it became apparent that this initiative must be ethnopharmacologic in order to increase the probability that only the most useful CNS agents are studied. It was also proposed that they must be extracted in the proper fashion in order to retain the active constituent(s); thus, not only should organic solvent extracts be evaluated, but also water-soluble extracts (such as those traditionally prepared as a tea). Professional American herbalists regard tinctures as the preferable formulation due to their high potency and long shelf life. A tincture is usually a 25 to 90% ethanol/water solution, depending on the particular plant (Wooding, 1994).

---

[5] Psychotherapeutic Drug Discovery and Development Program. PA-92-15. October 1991.
[6] International Cooperative Biodiversity Groups. RFA TW-92-01, June 1992.

The NIMH Screening Program

This screening program consists of a contract to facilitate the pharmacologic profiling of potential new drugs and natural products. The contract (currently with NovaScreen) provides state of-the-art in vitro assays for up to 100 different CNS receptors (Table 1) for facilitating the screening of potential new drugs. These assays are available to any scientist for the purpose of drug discovery and development. Initial studies with natural products were begun in 1991. The first step was to select some commercially available natural products extracts commonly used by North American herbalists for various CNS indications. These extracts were screened through the above-mentioned receptor binding assays. The results of these initial screens are shown in Table 2.

The high receptor affinity of these extracts suggests that a standard oral dose would be sufficient to produce a real pharmacologic effect in vivo (assuming that they are sufficiently bioavailable). The activity of *G biloba* (maidenhair tree) was not followed up by the NIMH, due to recent developments in Europe. While ginkgo has been available OTC in Europe for many years for the treatment of cerebral insufficiency, a standardized leaf extract (from Schwabe GmbH; called EGb 761) was approved by the German BGA in July 1994 for use in dementia (Bundes Anzeiger, 1994). Comprehensive aspects of the pharmacology and therapeutic effects of this valuable medicinal plant are found in other sections of this book and in Itil and Martorano (1995). Germany currently licenses formulations from several other herbals; see Table 2.[7] Hops are used for anxiety and sleep disorders, passion flower for nervous unrest, and valerian for insomnia (its safety profile includes a lack of synergy with ethanol).[8] The activity of one plant, Saint-John's-wort, is summarized in the following.

Hypericum Perforatum (Saint John'swort)

Hypericum perforatum was chosen as an example of a medicinal plant that has been used for centuries (typically prepared as a tea or as an olive oil extract) for various medical purposes, including depression (Murray, 1992; Hobbs, 1989). A clinical trial with this plant was carried out in Germany (Muldner & Zoller, 1984).[9]

---

[7] German Ministry of Health. Commission E. Monographs for Phytomedicines. Bonn, Germany: German Ministry of Health, 1985.

[8] ESCOP, European Scientific Cooperative for Phytotherapy. Valerian root. Meppel, The Netherlands: European Scientific Cooperative for Phytotherapy, 1990.

[9] Since the presentation of this paper, several publications evaluating the effects of hypericum in depression have appeared. For a recent meta-analysis of the German studies, see Linde et al., 1996.

TABLE 1.

NIMH/NovaScreen Receptor Binding/Enzyme Activity Assays

Amino Acids	
Quisqualate	Glycine (nonstrychnine)
Kainate	Glycine (strychnine)
MK-801	$GABA_A$, $GABA_B$
NMDA	Benzodiazepine
PCP	Sigma
Biogenic Amines*	
Adrenergic ($\alpha_{1,2}, \beta$)	Serotonin ($5\text{-}HT_{1A,1B,1C,2,3}$)
Dopamine (DA_{1-4})	Histamine (H_1, H_2)
Muscarinic (M_{1-3})	
Peptides	
Angiotensin II	Arg-Vasopressin 1
Bombesin	CCK_A, CCK_B
Neurokinin (NK1, NK2)	Substance K
Neurotensin	Neuropeptide Y
VIP	Somatostatin
Peptide Factors	Channel Proteins
ANF	Calcium (N, T, L)
NGF	Chloride
EGF	Potassium
Second Messengers	Miscellaneous
Forskolin	Adenosine (A1, A2)
Phorbol ester	Opiate (nonselective)
Inositol triphosphate	AIDS (e.g., gp 120)
Enzyme Assays	
Acetyl CoA synthetase	Protein kinase C
Leukotriene A_4 hydrolase	Acetylcholinesterase
Leukotriene C_4 synthetase	MAO_A, MAO_B

* Initial ligands nonselective followed by selective for subtype

TABLE 2.

Receptor Binding Activity of Some Commercial Extracts*

Plant name	Reported CNS activity (traditional use)	Receptors with $K_i \leq 2$ μg crude extract/ml
Ginkgo biloba (ginkgo)	PAF antagonist, antioxidant, anti-inflammatory (senility, asthma, vascular disorders)	GABA$_A$, GABA$_B$, AMPA, kainate, CCK$_A$
Valeriana officinalis (valerian)	Sedative, hypnotic, antispasmodic, carminative (insomnia, intestinal colic, antidepressant)	GABA$_B$, AMPA, kainate, NMDA, CCK$_A$
Passiflora incarnata (passion flower)	Sedative, hypnotic, antispasmodic (insomnia)	GABA$_A$, GABA$_B$, AMPA, glycine, NMDA, Cl$^-$
Matricaria chamomilla (German chamomile)	Sedative, antispasmodic, anti-inflammatory (insomnia, neuralgia, lumbago, rashes,)	GABA$_A$, GABA$_B$, AMPA, kainate, glycine, NMDA, CCK$_A$, Cl$^-$
Humulus lupulus (hops)	Sedative, antiseptic, astringent (anxiety, insomnia)	GABA$_A$, GABA$_B$, AMPA, kainate, glycine, NMDA, CCK$_{A,B}$, Cl$^-$
Nepeta cataria (catnip)	Aromatic, antispasmodic, anodyne (upset stomach, diarrhea, bronchitis, insomnia)	GABA$_A$, GABA$_B$, AMPA, kainate, NMDA, CCK$_A$, Cl$^-$
Hypericum perforatum (Saint John's wort)	Inhibits MAO, antiviral, antidepressant (depression, anxiety, insomnia)	GABA$_A$, GABA$_B$, adenosine
Centella asiatica (gotu kola)	Antibiotic, ↑ hyaluronic acid and chondroitinsulfate (nerve tonic, skin problems, antiaging)	Glycine, CCK$_A$

* Sources include: Murray and Pizzorno, 1991; Lust, 1974; Mowrey, 1990; Hoffmann, 1992.

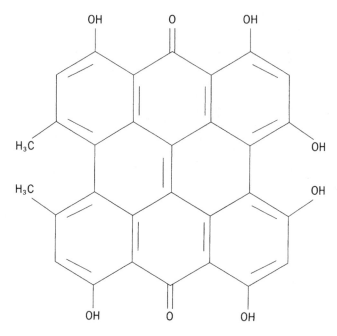

Figure 1. Hypericin.

In 6 women with depressive symptoms the effect on the excretion of urinary metabolites of noradrenaline and dopamine was measured after a monotherapy with the active hypericin complex (Psychotonin M). In all patients there was a significant increase in 3-methoxy-4-hydroxyphenyl glucol, which was considered an expression of a beginning antidepressive effect. When the same patients were supplemented with further 9 cases, the clinical influence on the depression was measured during a period of 4-6 weeks using the rating-scales SCAG (Clinical Assessment Geriatric Scale) and DSI (Depression Status Inventory), there was a quantitative improvement in the items: anxiety, dysphoric mood, loss of interest, hypersomnia, anorexia, depression regularly worse in the morning, insomnia, obstipation, psychomotoric retardation and feeling of worthlessness.

Hypericum has been known since the 1950s to contain a pigment, hypericin (Fig. 1). While most contemporary pharmacognosists assume that hypericin is

TABLE   3.

Receptor Binding Activity of *Hypericum perforatum* Crude Extract

Extract Concentration (μg/ml)	% Inhibition in Various Assays							
	Adenosine	$GABA_A$	$GABA_B$	$5HT_1$	BDZ	IP_3	MAO_A	MAO_B
0.005	−2	7	45	12	−4	−3	9	−1
0.05	13	43	85	12	0	16	4	−10
0.5	17	94	105	9	0	13	33	−2
5.0	20	100	109	12	19	40	97	53
50	71	101	114	54	65	107	—	—
∼K_i (μg/ml)*	1	0.075	0.006	25	24	10	2	3.2

$* K_i = / C_{50} / 1 + ligand\ affinity / ligand\ concentration$

TABLE   4.

Receptor Binding Activity of Hypericin

Concentration (μM)	*% Inhibition*		
	MAO_A	MAO_B	*NMDA*
0.001	—	—	10.5
0.01	—	—	24.5
0.1	—	—	−0.3
1	—	—	48.5
10	27.0	−2.0	81.7
100	20.8	−20.7	—
∼K_1	—	—	1.1

the primary active compound in this plant genus, detailed pharmacologic data are lacking. Other important constituents of several species of *Hypericum* include flavonoids, xanthones, phenolic carboxylic acids, essential oils, carotenoids, alkanes, and phloroglucinol derivatives (Murray, 1992).

A commercially available extract containing ∼0.1% hypericin was dried under vacuum, dissolved in 4% dimethy sulfoxide (DMSO), and diluted to assay concentrations of 0.005 to 50 μg/ml. Results from a battery of 39 receptor assays and two enzyme inhibition assays are shown in Table 3.

Hypericin (95%, Sigma) was found to lack MAO_A or MAO_B inhibition at concentrations up to 10 μM (Table 4). This is in contrast to a previous report that hypericin did inhibit MAO (IC_{50}∼100 μM or 50 μg/ml ; Suzuki et al., 1984). One possible explanation is that the hypericin used by Suzuki et al. was an extract of only 80% purity. It is possible that one or more constituents of the

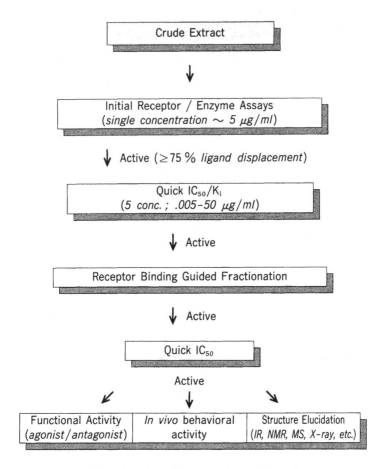

Figure 2. Flowchart for screening CNS active compounds from natural products.

remaining 20% of this preparation could account for this enzyme inhibition and would thus be consistent with the present finding. Hypericin, which did show activity at the NMDA receptor ($K_i \sim 1 \mu M$), is currently in early clinical trials in the United States as an antiviral (Meruelo et al., 1988). This NMDA activity may be important for its reported antiviral activity.

STUDIES OF MEDICINAL PLANTS BASED ON AYURVEDA

A collaborative effort to identify and develop antiaging, memory-enhancing drugs was developed in 1990 with Dr. Sukh Dev of the Indian Institute of

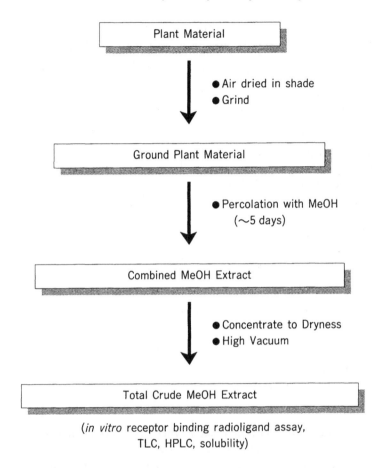

(*in vitro* receptor binding radioligand assay,
TLC, HPLC, solubility)

Figure 3. General extraction scheme for Ayurvedic
crude drugs.

Technology in New Delhi. This consists of screening crude plant extracts based
on "Ayurveda" and Ayurvedic crude drugs used in the traditional system of
medicine in India. More than 100 plant samples and several Ayurvedic drugs
(Rasayan) were collected and extracted in cold methanol for screening. A
systematic scheme for evaluating these plant extracts was devised and is illus-
trated in Figure 2. The basic extraction scheme is shown in Figure 3.

Several crude extracts and fractions have shown significant initial receptor
activity in assays, which may be related to their purported effects on memory and
longevity. They are summarized in Table 5.

Of interest with these plants is that fractionation does not result in increased

TABLE 5.

Receptor Binding Studies on Ayurvedic Crude Drugs

Plant name (part) MeOH extract fraction	*Receptor binding* $\sim K_i (\mu g/ml)$		
	$GABA_A$	$GABA_B$	CCK_A
Withania somnifera (root)	0.29	1.8	—
BuOH fraction	—	41	—
Aqueous fraction	0.37	5	—
Terminalia bellerica (fruit)	—	—	0.25
BuOH fraction	—	—	14
Ethyl acetate (EA) whole fraction	—	14	6
EA-1	—	—	9
EA-2	—	—	7
EA-3	—	—	6
EA-4	—	—	5
EA-5	—	—	10
EA-6*	—	—	—
EA-7*	—	—	—
EA-8*	—	—	—
EA-9*	—	—	—
EA-10*	—	—	1.6
EA-11*	—	—	1.5

* pure compound
— No significant binding

potency. In all cases thus far, *the crude extract has shown greater activity than the fractions*. Other investigators have reported similar results with crude extracts of *Withania somnifera*. Mehta et al. (1991) found that an MeOH extract inhibits γ-aminobutyric acid $(GABA_A)$ binding and TBPS (a Cl^- channel ligand) binding, as well as enhances benzodiazepine binding. Withanolides are steroidal compounds extracted from *W somnifera*. Two glycowithanolides, called sitoindosides IX and X, have been isolated and reported to have anxiolytic and memory-enhancing effects in mice and rats (Ghosal et al., 1989).

A visit to the National Institute of Mental Health and Neuro Science (NIMHANS) in Bangalore, India, by a delegation from the United States in 1993 provided the stimulus for additional experiments. Investigators there have been actively examining the utility of Ayurvedic preparations for schizophrenia (Mahal et al., 1976; Ramu et al., 1992). The initial study consisted of four treatment groups:

1. *Brahmyadiyoga* (a mixture of six plants: *Acorus calamus*, *Centella asiatica*, *Nardostachys jatamansi*, *Rauwolfia serpentina*, *Saussurea lappa*, and

Valeriana wallichii). Dosage was 8 to 12g divided into four doses.
2. *Tagara* (valerian alone). Dosage was 8 to 12g divided into four doses.
3. Chlorpromazine (200 to 300 mg/day).
4. Placebo.

Some explanation regarding the Ayurvedic System of medicine is probably in order. In this system, 28 different types of *ummada* (schizophrenia) are described. The usual treatment consists of three parts: *daivavyapashraya chikitsa* or spiritual therapy, *satwavajaya chikitsa* or psychotherapy, and *yuktivyapashraya chikitsa* or physical medicine, which normally includes both drugs and a special diet. To reduce the number of variables in this study, the authors used only the drug treatment. The six plants contained in the primary treatment are for different purposes; not all of them are used for psychosis. In Western terminology, saussurea is used for epilepsy, nardostachys for depression and anxiety, acorus and valerian as sedatives (acorus has been used by itself with some success), and centella as a tonic (this plant is used for almost everything). The authors describe the mixture as an: "anticonvulsant, increases memory, tranquilizes the overactivity of brain cells, a sedative and hypnotic, an antipsychotic, and a brain tonic."

That said, of 108 patients completing a two-month treatment, the investigators found that the six-plant combination was significantly more effective (as measured by a standard Western psychiatric scale) than placebo and not significantly different from chlorpromazine. Valerian alone produced no significant improvement (Mahal et al., 1976).

The discerning pharmacologist might conclude that the reserpine content in the rauwolfia accounts for the antipsychotic activity. This idea was tested by determining the receptor binding characteristics of a crude methanol extract of rauwolfia and the other plants in *Brahmyadiyoga*. The results are shown in Table 6.

The high affinity of the rauwolfia extract for the α_2 and D_2 receptors was somewhat surprising. Reserpine would not be expected to have this activity since reserpine is thought to act on catecholamine and serotonin storage vesicles, depleting these amines. This binding may be of importance. Adrenergic receptor binding is probably due to the presence of yohimbine, a structurally related compound that is also found in rauwolfia. Investigators in the NIMH intramural program found that the addition of an α_2 antagonist, idazoxan, to fluphenazine in schizophrenic patients augments the therapeutic effect (Litman et al., 1993). Considerable α_2 binding was also seen by this same group in its studies of Korean medicinal plants used in the treatment of psychoses (two of which are the same as those used here: acorus and saussurea) (Chung et al., 1995). In China, rauwolfia is used as a sedative, as an antihypertensive, and as a treatment for

TABLE 6.

Receptor Binding Studies on *Brahmyadiyoga**

Plant name (part) MeOH extract	Receptor binding~K_i (μg/ml)		
	α_2	D_2	GABA$_B$
Rauwolfia serpentina (root)	1.4	1.5	27.3
Centella asiatica (leaves)	—	—	21
Saussurea lappa (root)	—	—	—
Acorus calamus (root)	—	—	—
Nordostachys jatamansi (root)	—	—	—
Valeriana wallichii (root)	—	—	—

* less than 75 % displacement at 50 μg/ml shown as " — "

snake-bite; saussurea is used as a tonic and stimulant, among other things (Duke & Ayensu, 1985).

Another finding of potential significance is the activity of many of these plants at GABA receptors. GABA agonists have been shown to inhibit the effects of direct or indirect acting dopamine agonists (Cott et al., 1976; Cott & Engel, 1977). The GABA$_B$ receptor agonist baclofen (Frederiksen, 1975) and the GABA analog γ-hydroxybutyrate (Schulz et al., 1981) were reported to have positive effects in schizophrenia, although subsequent reports have failed to confirm this finding (Simpson et al., 1976; Lloyd & Morsell, 1987). In addition, chronically administered GABA agonists result in enhanced functional activity and increased numbers of serotonin receptors (Green et al., 1985; Metz et al., 1985).

While the lack of binding activity at any of the 40 receptors for four of these plants is surprising, other pharmacologic activities that are not included in this screen should also be examined before abandoning the search.[10] Screens designed on the basis of known mechanisms and sites of action will not reveal the existence of compounds having novel modes of action.

DISCUSSION

Herbs have been consumed by human beings for hundreds or even thousands of years; WHO has estimated that 88% of the world's population rely chiefly on traditional medicine (Farnsworth et al., 1985). On March 13, 1992, WHO released its *Guidelines for the Assessment of Herbal Medicines* (Akerele, 1992). These guidelines represent a major step in a standardization of the way developed countries can incorporate traditional medicines into modern health care systems. Olaylwola Akerele. M.D., former director of WHO's Traditional Medicine

---

[10] The identity of these latter 4 extracts is now in question.

Program, points out that "the guidelines can be regarded as the first *official* guidance for health authorities, industry, academic community, and other interested parties for the assessment of herbal medicines and can, later on, be adopted for the assessment of other natural products" (McCaleb, 1994).

The essence of these guidelines is that the historical use of a substance is a valid form of safety and efficacy information, in the absence of scientific documentation to the contrary. With regard to safety, the guidelines say:

> A guiding principle should be that, if the product has been traditionally used without demonstrated harm, no specific restrictive regulatory actions should be undertaken unless new evidence demands a revised risk-benefit assessment... Prolonged and apparently uneventful use of a substance usually offers testimony of its safety.

With respect to efficacy, the guidelines say:

> For treatment of minor disorders and for nonspecific indications, some relaxation is justified in the requirements for proof of efficacy, taking into account the extent of traditional use; the same considerations may apply to prophylactic use.

The documented use of sophisticated phytomedicinals by such advanced countries as Germany, France, and Japan has resulted in a wealth of documentation and clinical experience. Some of these products have been used by millions of Europeans under clinical supervision. Legislators, the public, and the medical communities in the United States are beginning to take note of these countries whose citizens pay a fraction of our health care costs, and in many cases enjoy better health. In Germany, products such as standardized ginkgo are regulated by a monograph system. Approval of such medicines requires more scientific documentation than for herbal remedies, but far less than the U.S. new drug approval process. The German Commission E monographs provide a good example of how the United States might simplify the approval of natural products at a reasonable cost and without sacrificing standards of safety or quality. In the absence of regulatory guidelines in the United States, private research organizations interested in this area have been making some significant progress. There are approximately 400 major herbs in commerce in the United States today. Of these, 279 have been approved by the FDA as safe food

---

[11]Herb Research Foundation, 1007 Pearl St., Suite 200, Boulder, CO80302.
[12]American Botanical Council, P.O. Box 201660, Austin, TX 78720-1660.

ingredients. For the remaining 121, the Herb Research Foundation[11] has conducted professional safety evaluations of 25 and plans to research another 40 in the next two years (McCaleb, 1994). Other organizations actively involved in scientific research with herbals include the American Botanical Council[12] and the American Herbal Products Association.

Botanicals are very diverse as consumer products, ranging from simple conventional foods, such as chamomile and peppermint, to products with potent pharmacologic activity, such as rauwolfia (from which reserpine is derived) and foxglove (from which digitalis is derived). This range of activity requires a flexible regulatory mechanism to address safety and efficacy in a responsible way without requiring the costly research necessary for new chemical entities. Most countries outside the United States have found ways to accommodate traditional medicines as well as the more sophisticated phytomedicinals safely and with apparent public health benefits that the United States has failed to realize. The United States should consider the adoption of a similar registration process to encourage new drug development in this country.

REFERENCES

Akerele, A. (1992): WHO guidelines for the assessment of herbal medicines. *Fitoterapia* **62** (2), 99-110. Summarized in *Herbalgram* **28**, 13-20, 1993.

Blumenthal, M. (1992): German MDs required to pass herb exam. *Herbalgram* **26**, 45.

Bundes Anzeiger (Federal Register of Germany) (1994), No. 133, Vla /414.

Cade, J.F.J. (1949): Lithium salts in the treatment of psychotic excitement. *Med. J. Aus.* **2**, 349-352.

Carlsson, A. (1959): The occurrence, distribution and physiological role of catecholamines in the nervous system. *Pharmacol. Rev.*, **11**, 490.

Carlsson, A., Lindqvist, M. (1963): Effect of chlorpromazine and haloperidol on formation of 3-methoxytyramine and normetanephrine in mouse brain. *Acta Pharmacol. Toxicol.*, **20**, 140.

Chung, I.-W., Kim, Y.-S., Ahn, J.-S., et al. (1995): Pharmacologic profile of natural products used to treat psychotic illnesses. *Psychopharm. Bull.*, **31**, 139-145.

Cott, J. (1994): U.S. efforts in natural products research. In: *INDO-U.S. Symposium on the Decade of the Brain*, Bangalore, India, February 8-14, 1993.

Cott, J., Carlsson, A., Engel, J., Lindqvist, M. (1976): Suppression of ethanol-induced locomotor stimulation by GABA-like drugs. *Naunyn Schmiedebergs Arch. Pharmacol.* **295** (3), 203-209.

Cott, J.M., Engel, J. (1977): Suppression by GABAergic drugs of the locomotor stimulation induced by morphine, amphetamine, and apomorphine: evidence for both pre- and post-synaptic inhibition of catecholamine systems. *J. Neural Transm.* **40** (4), 253-268.

Dastur, J.F. (1960): *Everybody's Guide to Ayurvedic Medicine*. Bombay, India: Taraporevala.

Dorfman, L., Furlenmeier, A., Huebner, C.F., et al. (1954): On the constitution of reserpine from Rauwolfia serpintina Benth. *Helv. Chim. Acta.* **37**, 368-369.

Duke, J.A., Ayensu, E.S. (1985): *Medicinal Plants of China*. Algonac, MI: Reference Publications.

Eisenberg, D.M., Kessler, R.C., Foster, C., et al. (1993): Unconventional medicine in the United States: Prevalence, costs, and patterns of use. *N. Engl. J. Med.* **328**, 246-252.

Farnsworth, N.R., Akerele, O., Bingel, A.S., et al. (1985): Medicinal plants in therapy. *Bull. WHO* **63** (6), 965-981,

Frederiksen, P.K. (1975): Baclofen in the treatment of schizophrenia. *Lancet* **1**, 702.

Ghosal, S., Lal, J., Srivastava, R., et al. (1989): Immunomodulatory and CNS effects of sitoindosides IX and X, two new glycowithanolides from *Withania somnifera. Phytother. Res.* **3** (5), 201-206.

Green, A.R., Johnson. P., Mountford, J.A., Nimgaonkar, V.L. (1985): Some anticonvulsant drugs alter monoamine-mediated behaviour in mice in ways similar to electroconvulsive shock; implications for antidepressant therapy. *Br. J. Pharmacol.* **84**, 337.

Haigler, H., Cott, J.M., Rudorfer, M., et al. (1993): Psychotherapeutic medications development program (PMDP). *Psychopharm. Bull.* **29** (2), 241-247.

Hobbs, C. (1989): St. John's wort, *Hypericum perforatum L. HerbalGram* **18/19**, 24-33.

Hoffman, D (1992): *The New Holistic Herbal*. Rockport, MA: Element.

Itil, T. Martorano, D. (1995): Natural substances in psychiatry (*Ginkgo biloba* in dementia). *Psychopharmacol. Bull.* **31** (1), 147-158.

Kline, N.S. (1954): Use of *Rauwolfia serpentina Benth.* in neuropsychiatric conditions. *Ann. N.Y. Acad. Sci.*, **59**, 107.

Kline, N.S. (1958): Clinical experience with iproniazid (Marsilid). *J. Clin. Exp. Psychopathol.* **19**, (suppl), 72-78.

Kuhn, R. (1958): The treatment of depressive states with G-22355 (imipramine hydrochloride). *Am. J. Psychiatry* **115**, 459-464.

Lehmann, H.E., Hanrahan, G.E. (1954): *AMA Arch. Neurol. Psychiatry* **71**, 227-237.

Linde, K. et al. (1996): St. John's wort for depression—an overview and meta-analysis of randomized clinical trials. *British Medical Journal* 313: 253-258.

Litman, R.E., Hong, W.W., Weissman, E.M., et al. (1993): Idazoxan, an α_2 antagonist, augments fluphenazine in schizophrenic patients: A pilot study. *J. Clin. Psychopharmacol.* **13**, 264-267.

Lloyd, K.G., Morselli, P.L. (1987): Psychopharmacology of GABAergic Drugs. In: F. Bloom (Ed.). *Psychopharmacology: The third generation of progress*. New York: Raven Press. 183-195.

Loomer, H.P., Saunders J.C., Kline, N.S. (1957): A clinical and pharmacodynamic evaluation of iproniazid as a psychic energizer. *Psychiat. Res. Rep.* **8**, 129-141.

Lust, J. (1974): *The Herb Book*. New York: Bantam.

Mahal, A.S., Ramu, N.G., Chaturvedi, D.D., et al. (1976): Double blind controlled study of brahmyadiyoga and tagara in the management of various types of unmada (schizophrenia). *Indian J. Psychiat.* **18**, 283–292.

McCaleb, R.S. (1994): Safety and regulation of herbal products. *Proceedings*, 5th Annual Symposium of the American Herbalists Guild, pp. 78–82.

Mehta, A.K., Binkley, P., Gandhi, S.S., Ticku, M.K. (1991): Pharmacologic effects of *Withania somnifera* root extract on GABA_A receptor complex. *Indian J. Med. Res.* (B) **94**, 312–315.

Meruelo, D., et al. (1988): Therapeutic agents with dramatic antiretroviral activity and little toxicity at effective doses: Aromatic polycyclic diones hypericin and pseudohypericin. *Proc. Nat. Acad. Sci.* **85**, 5230–5234.

Metz, A., Goodwin, G.M., Green, A.R. (1985): The administration of baclofen to mice increases $5-HT_2$-mediated head-twitch behaviour and 5-HT receptor number in frontal cortex. *Neuropharmacology* **24**, 357.

Mowrey, D.B. (1990): *Next Generation Herbal Medicine*. New Canaan, CT: Keats.

Muldner, V.H., Zoller, M. (1984): Antidepressive wirkung eines auf den wirkstoffkomplex hypericin standardisierten hypericum-extrakes. (Antidepressive effect of a Hypericum extract standardized to an active hypericin complex. Biochemical and clinical studies). *Arzneim Forsch.* **34**, 918–920.

Müller, J.M., Schlitter, E., Bein, H.J. (1952): Reserpine. *Experientia* **8**, 338.

Murray, M.T., Pizzorno, J.E. (1991): *Encyclopedia of Natural Medicine*. Rocklin, CA: Prima.

Murray, M.T. (1992): St. John's wort (*Hypericum perforatum*). In: *The Healing Power of Herbs*. Rocklin, CA: Prima.

Ramu, M.G., Venkataram, B.S., Mukundan, H., et al. (1992): A controlled study of Ayurvedic treatment in the acutely ill patients with schizophrenia (Unmāda) — Rationale and results. *NIMHANS J.* **10** (1), 1–16.

Rush, B. (1774): *An Inquiry Into the Natural History of Medicine Among the Indians of North America, and a Comparative View of Their Diseases and Remedies with Those of Civilized Nations*. Philadelphia: American Philosophical Society.

Schulz, S.C.H., Van Kammen, D.P., Buchsbaum, M.S., et al. (1981): γ-Hydroxybutyrate treatment of schizophrenia: A pilot study. *Pharmacopsychiatry* **14**, 129.

Selikoff, I.J., Robitzek, E.H., Ornstein, G.G. (1952): Toxicity of hydrazine derivatives of isonicotinic acid in the chemotherapy of human tuberculosis. *Q. Bull. Seaview Hosp.* **13**, 17–26.

Sen, G., Bose, K.C. (1931): Rauwolfia serpentina. *Indian Med. World*, **2**, 194.

Simpson, G.M., Branchey, M.H., Shrivastava, R.K. (1976): Baclofen in schizophrenia. *Lancet* **1**, 1245.

Soejarto, D.D., Farnsworth, N.R. (1939): Tropical rainforests: Potential sources of new drugs? *Perspect. Biol. Med.* **32** (2), 244–256.

Suzuki, O., Katsumata, Y., Oya, M., Wagner, H. (1984): Inhibition of monoamine oxidase by hypericin. *Planta Med.* **50**, 272–274.

Wooding, R. (1994): Methods of preparation. *Proceedings*, 5th Annual Symposium of the American Herbalists Guild, p. 100.

6

Indian Medicinal Plants as a Source of CNS Active Drugs*

B.N. Dhawan

The exploitation of Indian medicinal plants saw a spurt of activity following the introduction of reserpine from Rauwolfia serpentina *to psychiatric practice. Although no new drug has been marketed, several promising leads have been obtained and some of them are being developed further.*

A central nervous system (CNS) depressant activity has been obtained more frequently than a stimulant activity. Jatamansone, a sesquiterpene lactone from the essential oil of Nardostachys jatamansi, *has been evaluated clinically, as well as experimentally, for neuroleptic activity. Asarone, isolated from* Acorus calamus, *appears to be a promising neuroleptic in experimental studies. Analgesic activity has been reported in several plants, and CNS stimulant and antidepressant constituents have also been isolated from a few plants.*

The Central Drug Research Institute (CDRI) has screened about 4000 taxonomically authenticated terrestrial plant materials and about 800 marine products for a wide variety of CNS depressant and stimulant effects. Active constituents have been isolated from several plants showing CNS depressant activity, but the most promising lead appears to be bacosides from Bacopa monniera *as a nootropic agent. Clinical studies are in progress with this product.*

Many clinically useful drugs that act on the CNS (morphine, ephedrine, hyoscine, caffeine, etc.), as well as drugs of abuse (mescaline, marijuana) have been isolated from plants. The natural products have initiated several new groups

---

*Presented at the Symposium on Development of CNS Active Agents from Plants of the 19th CINP Congress, June 27-July 1, 1994, Washington, D.C.

of neuropharmacologic agents, the most recent example being the development of psychotropic drugs following the introduction of reserpine. This has not been followed by an increased global effort to exploit natural products, which is partly attributable to the increased cost of new drug discovery and the industry's wish to have strong patent protection in order to recover the cost. The interest had been maintained in selected plants, a notable example being *Ginkgo biloba* (Braquet, 1988). Similarly, a substantial amount of work has been done on the cannabinoids (Rapaka & Makriyannis, 1987) and with the diterpene coleonol (Dubey et al., 1974), which is also known as forskolin (Bhatt et al., 1977), and whose major use has been as a neuropharmacologic tool (Seamon et al., 1981). The recent revival of interest in this area has major commercial considerations. Thus, natural products represent a renewable resource; the technology is environmentally friendly; the products have better patient acceptance and tolerance (Dhawan, 1995); and, above all, the molecular diversity in natural products continues to be a major source of new lead generation (Hylands & Nisbet, 1991).

Indian investigators, however, have continued to study a large number of plants for their potential CNS effects, even though, in most cases, the studies have been rather fragmentary or preliminary in nature. Very few concerted or well-coordinated efforts have been made to develop new drugs, except for the work done in the author's own laboratory (which will be summarized later). The recent work done in India has been described elsewhere (Satyavati, 1984; Dhawan, 1986; Patnaik & Dhawan, 1995). This chapter, therefore, includes only those plants on which detailed work has been done, in which a new type of activity has been uncovered, or from which active compounds have been isolated and characterized. Work on well-known natural products, such as rauwolfia alkaloids or cannabinoids, has not been included owing to space limitations. The plants are grouped according to the type of CNS activity involved.

ANALGESIC ACTIVITY

Several plants exhibited promising activity but active constituents have been isolated from only a few. Vohora et al. (1981) isolated 2α, 3β, 20β-Ur-2en-23β-28 dioic acid 3-diacetate from *Corchorus depressus*. It has analgesic and antipyretic activity, but does not produce CNS depression. Several glycosides have been cbtained from related species of *Corchorus* but have not been biologically evaluated (Rastogi & Mehrotra, 1993). Palanicharry and Nagrajan (1990) have demonstrated significant analgesic activity in kaempferol 3-o-sophoroside from the leaves of *Cassia alata*. A pterocarpinoid gangetin, isolated from the roots of *Desmodium gangeticum* (Ghosh & Anand Kumar, 1983), as well as oleanolic acid 3-β-glucostide, isolated from *Randia dumetorium* seed (Ghosh et al., 1983), also showed significant analgesic action. Analgesic activity has also been reported in oleanolic acid isolated from *Luffa cylindrica* (Singh et al., 1992). Swertiamarin from *Swrertia purpurascens* (*S ciliata*) has been found to raise the pain threshold in mice for prolonged periods (Rastogi & Mehrotra, 1993).

A few plants have exhibited a morphine type of analgesic activity and deserve more in-depth studies to delineate their potentiality. Most detailed studies have been performed by Atal et al. (1984), with potassium embelate derived from *Embelia ribes*. The analgesic activity by the oral as well as the parenteral route was comparable to that of morphine. Morphine like analgesic activity has also been reported with gossipin obtained from *Gossypium indicum* (Vishwanathan et al., 1985). An interesting observation was the lack of development of tolerance on repeated administration.

ANTICONVULSANT ACTIVITY

Comparatively few plant constituents have exhibited anticonvulsant action. It is also difficult to compare results of different investigations because the parameters for producing convulsions are not identical. Total alkaloids of *Erythrina variegata* have anticonvulsant action without associated CNS depression (Ghosal et al., 1972). Most of the other reported compounds also produce CNS depression, and, therefore, the activity dose not appear to be specific. Such compounds include fumariline from *Fumaria indica* (Kumar et al., 1986), gindarine from *Stephania glabra* (Madan et al., 1974), xanthone glucoside from *S purpurascens* (Ghosal et al., 1974), and anglicin from *Selenium vaginatum* (Chandoke & Ray Ghatak, 1976). Further, some plants exhibiting tranquilizing activity also protect against experimental seizures; these are discussed under tranquilizers.

TRANQUILIZING ACTIVITY

Perhaps the most promising lead in this area after reserpine has been the α- and β- asarones from *A calamus*, whose pharmacology was reviewed by Dandiya & Sakina (1989). The compounds exhibit the classic effects of neuroleptic agents, such as hypothermia, the blockade of conditioned avoidance response, and a reduction in spontaneous motor activity. They also exhibit anticonvulsant activity. Asarones are, however, devoid of antiemetic activity and, unlike reserpine, do not deplete monoamines. Unfortunately, no developmental work has been undertaken on these compounds. Arora and his colleagues have done an impressive amount of work on the sesquiterpene ketone jatamansone from *N jatamansi* (summarized by Arora, 1985). The tranquilizing activity appears to be mediated via a serotonergic mechanism. It has mild sedative and anticonvulsant activity as well. A preliminary clinical trial in a few hyperkinetic children has been reported (Arora et al., 1966). A major limiting factor appears to be the hypotension observed in anesthetized as well as unanesthetized animals. Much less work has been done on the other reported compounds. Fumariline has been reported to have tranquilizing activity in addition to its anticonvulsant activity. The essential oils of *Blumea lacera* (Dixit & Varma 1976), *Cymopogon citratus* (Seth et al., 1976), and *Hedychium* species (Dixit & Varma, 1979), and *l*-nuciferine from *Nelumbo nucifera* (Bhattacharya et al., 1978b), which is also a dopamine receptor antagonist and has a chlorpromazine-like neuropharmacologic profile and gentianine from *Swertia chirayita* (Bhattacharya et al., 1974) also exhibit tranquilizing activity. Sheth et al. (1963) had reported good tranquilizing activity in a fraction from oil of *Celastrus paniculatus*, but the active constituent has not been isolated and characterized. More recently, it has been shown to facilitate learning (Karanth et al., 1980, 1981).

NONSPECIFIC CNS DEPRESSANT ACTIVITY

A number of natural products have been chemically characterized, but the CNS effects have not been well studied and they have been variously reported to have CNS depressant, sedative, or antianxiety effects. Several of them decrease motor activity and potentiate barbiturate hypnosis. Because of space constraints, a brief mention of only the more promising compounds will be made. It has been pointed out in the review of anticonvulsant compounds that several of them also show CNS depressant activity. Other important compounds from Indian plants with CNS depressant activity include xanthone calophylloide from *Calophyllum inophyllum* and mesuaxanthone A, B, and euxanthone from *Mesua ferrea* (Gopalkrishnan et al., 1980), essential oil of *Luvunga scandens* (Mishra & Agarwal, 1988), alkaloids of *Stephania wightii* (Nazimuddin et al., 1980), and tylophorine from *Tylophora indica* (Gopalkrishnan et al., 1979).

CNS STIMULANTS

The number of plants showing CNS stimulant activity has been much smaller. The plants have mainly exhibited monoamine oxidase (MAO) inhibitory, antidepressant, anerexigenic, or respiratory stimulant activity. *Alstonia scholaris* has yielded several interesting alkaloids. Among these, strictamine exhibits MAO inhibitory activity in vivo in mice and in vitro in rat brain and mitochondria, in addition to antidepressant activity (Bhattacharya et al., 1978a). Interestingly, the plant also yields another alkaloid picerinine that produces CNS depression (Dutta et al., 1976), as well as reserpine. Over 20 alkaloids have been obtained from a related species, *Alstonia venenata* (reviewed by Chatterji et al., 1978). Among these, alstovenine and ectiovetidine have been shown to inhibit MAO (Dhawan & Rastogi, 1991). Moreover, CNS stimulant activity has been reported in indolealkylamines from *Mucuna pruriens* (Rastogi & Mehrotra, 1991). Anorexigenic activity has been reported in alkaloids isolated from the fruits of *Melia azaderach* (Srivastava et al., 1981) and from the seeds of *Strychnos potatorum* (Singh & Kapoor, 1980).

MISCELLANEOUS ACTIVITIES

Gindarinine from *Stephania glabra* has been shown by Mahatma et al. (1987) to have local anesthetic activity in 1% concentration when used for infiltration and nerve block. Local anesthetic activity has also been reported in *Euphorbia nerifolia* (Lahon et al., 1979) and *Zizyphus jujuba* (Sahu & Das, 1975), but none of these have been followed up. Jamwal et al. (1962) have investigated in detail the central respiratory stimulant activity of osthol isolated from *Prangos pabularia*. Recently, Kulkarni and Verma (1992) reported the ability of an herbal preparation to attenuate the development of tolerance to morphine.

THE CDRI EXPERIENCE

A broad-based program of biologic screening of medicinal plants was initiated at CDRI in 1963 and the study of CNS effects forms an important part of this program. The data on about 3000 plants were reviewed a few years ago (Rastogi et al., 1987), and, to date, over 4000 taxonomically authenticated plant materials and about 800 marine organisms have been screened. The CNS test screen annually handles about 1000 test materials of varying grades of purity, starting with an initial 50% ethanolic extract. The activity is confirmed in one of the primary fractions before selecting a plant for detailed study. A battery of 11 tests in mice has been organized in four complementary modules, and details of the tests, as well as the organization of the program, have been published (Dhawan, 1991). Briefly, it involves the study of acute toxicity; the effect on gross behavior, drug interaction studies; some additional tests for such specific activities as analgesia, anticonvulsant activity, and so on; and a limited number of confirmatory tests in other species, such as rats (e.g., conditioned avoidance response) or cats (polysynaptic reflexes). About 2.6% of the plant extracts and 2% of the marine products exhibited confirmed CNS depressant activity. No stimulants were obtained from the plants, but 6.5% of the marine extracts had stimulant effects (Dhawan, 1995). About a dozen plants are being followed up, and chemical compounds from several of them have been isolated and characterized. These include diterpene conyzic acid (Sen et al., 1975), also called strictic acid (Tandon & Rastogi, 1979), and the flavone conyzatin (Tandon & Rastogi, 1979), and several other flavanoids from *Conyza stricta*, a pentacyclic triterpene lactone from *Dillenia indica* (Bannerji et al., 1975), a tetranortriterpene dysobinin from

Dysoxylum binectariferum (Singh et al., 1976), queretanoic (3ϕ) caffeate from *Melianthus major* (Agarwal & Rastogi, 1976), and auriculoside from *Acacia auriculiformis* (Sahai et al., 1980). Auriculoside is the first flavan glycoside shown to have CNS depressant activity.

Neuromuscular blocking activity has been obtained in several groups of alkaloids. A number of bisbenzylisoquinoline alkaloids have been isolated from the roots of *Cissampelos pariera* (Dhawan & Rastogi, 1991). Among these, methiodide salt of hayatin (Bhattacharji et al., 1952) had potent neuromuscular blocking activity (Pradhan & De, 1953). In clinical studies, however, it produced a steep fall in blood pressure in some cases (Pradhan et al., 1964). A new abnormal erythrina alkaloid isococculidine from *Cocculus laurifolius* showed good neuromuscular blocking activity (Kar et al., 1977). Significant neuromuscular blocking activity was also exhibited by another quaternary alkaloid, isocorydine methochloride (Mukherjee et al., 1984). Both, however, failed to exhibit significant advantages over available neuromuscular blocking agents.

A useful approach employed by CDRI during the past 10 years has been the use of specific test systems for drugs used in Indian traditional systems of medicine. The most promising lead among the CNS active plants has been provided by *B monniera*, an herb used in Ayurveda for improving learning and memory (Chunekar, 1960). The crude extract of the plant enabled rats to have better acquisition and retention, coupled with delayed extinction, in acute as well as subacute paradigms of learning and memory (Singh & Dhawan, 1982). Subsequent detailed studies (Singh et al., 1988, 1990) showed these effects to be due to earlier isolated saponins, bacoside A (Chatterji et al., 1965) and bacoside B (Basu et al., 1967). The saponins facilitate both positive and negative reinforcement. They also prevent amnesia due to electroshock and stress (Singh & Dhawan, 1994) and prevent stress-induced increases in brain lipids (unpublished observations). Clinical studies have been initiated with the mixture of bacosides.

CONCLUSIONS AND FUTURE STRATEGIES

It is clear that a very large number of Indian plants has been studied, but there have been few coordinated efforts toward drug development. Further, in several cases, botanically unauthenticated plant materials have been used. Finally, the active plants are not always available in adequate quantity. In such cases, the active compounds represent good leads, and it is necessary to optimize them with synthetic or semisynthetic molecules.

India has a huge flora population, including a large number of endemic plants. However, information about only a limited number of plants is available in traditional systems of Indian medicine. It is, therefore, necessary to study most of remaining plants in a CDRI type of broad-based CNS screen. The marine flora also represent a rich resource which has been little investigated, and an exploration should prove rewarding.

The priority areas in which to develop new centrally acting agents should be drugs that affect learning and memory, psychotropic agents, and plants capable of affecting dependence liability or its management. It should also be necessary to consider the availability of plant material and the yield of active constituents before selecting such plants for a detailed study. Finally, more sensitive test systems, including in vitro screens, must be developed.

Indian scientists are aware of the potentialities of the country's rich terrestrial and marine flora, and several multidisciplinary efforts are being initiated. It is hoped that a number of new therapeutic agents for the treatment of CNS disorders will become available from Indian natural products during the next 5 to 10 years.

REFERENCES

Agarwal, J.S., Rastogi, R.P. (1976): Queretanoic (30) caffeate and other constituents of *Melianthus major*. *Phytochem*. **15**, 430-431.

Arora, R.B. (Ed.) (1985): *Development of Unani Drugs from Herbal Sources and the Role of Elements in Their Mechanism of Action*. p. 75. New Delhi: Hamdard National Foundation.

Arora, R.B., Chatterji, A.K., Gupta. R.D., et al. (1966): Neuropharmacological profile of jatamansone with special reference to its effectiveness in hyperkinetic states. In: G.S. Sidhu, I.K. Kackar, P.B. Sattur, et al. (Eds.), *CNS Drugs*, 118-132. New Delhi: Council of Scientific and Industrial Research.

Atal, C.K., Siddiqui, M.A., Zutshi, U., et al. (1984): Non-narcotic orally effective, centrally acting analgesic from an Ayurvedic drug. *J. Ethnopharmacol*. **11**, 309-317.

Banerji, N., Majumdar, R.C., Dutta, N.L. (1975): A new pentacyclic triterpene lactone from *Dillenia indica*. *Phytochem*. **14**, 1447-1448.

Basu, N., Rastogi, R.P., Dhar. M.L., (1967): Chemical examination of Bacopa monniera Wettst: Part 3—Bacoside B. *Ind. J. Chem*. **5**, 84-86.

Bhatt, S.V. Bajwa, B.S., Dornauer, H., deSouza, N.J. (1977): Structure and stereochemistry of new labdane diterpinoids from *Coleus forskohlii. Bri Tetrahedron Lett*. **19**, 1669-1672.

Bhattacharji, S., Sharma, V.N., Dhar, M.L. (1952): Chemical examination of the roots of *Cissampelos pareira. Linn. J. Sci. Indus. Res*. **11B**. 81-82.

Bhattacharya, S.K., Bose, R., Dutta. S.C., et al. (1978a): Neuropharmacological studies on strictamine isolated from *Alstonia scholaris. Ind. J. Exp. Biol*. **17**, 598-600.

Bhattacharya, S.K., Bose, R., Ghosh, P., et al. (1978b): Psychopharmacological studies on (-)-nuciferine and its Hofmann degradation product atherosperminine. *Psychopharmacology* **59**, 29-33.

Bhattacharya, S.K., Ghosal, S., Chaudhari, R.K., et al. (1974): Chemical constituents of Gentianaceae XI: Antipsychotic activity of Gentianine. *J. Pharmaceut. Sci*. **63**, 1341-1342.

Braquet, P., (Ed.) (1988): *Ginkgolides—Chemistry, Biology and Clinical Perspectives*, Vol. 1, 2. Barcelona: Prous.

Chandoke, N., Ray Ghatak, B.J. (1976): Pharmacological investigation of angelicin, a tranquillosedative and anticonvulsant agent. *Ind. J. Med. Res.* **63**, 833–841.

Chatterji, A., Mukhopadhyay, S., Ray, A.B. (1978): Alkaloids of *Alstonia venenata*. *J. Sci. Indus. Res.* **37**, 187–202.

Chatterji, N., Rastogi, R.P., Dhar, M.L. (1965): Chemical examination of *Bacopa monniera* Wettst. II—Constitution of bacoside A. *Ind. J. Chem.* **3**, 24–29.

Chunekar, K.C. (1960): *Hindi Translation of Bhav Prakash Nighantu*, p. 372. Varanasi: Chowkhamba Vidya Bhawan.

Dandiya, P.C., Sakina, M.R. (1989): CNS drugs: Work done and future strategies In: P.C. Dandiya, S.B. Vohora (Eds.). *Research and Development of Indigenous Drugs*. 34–44. New Delhi: Institute on History of Medicine and Medical Research.

Dhawan, B.N. (Ed.) (1986): *Current Research on Medicinal Plants in India*. New Delhi: Indian National Science Academy.

Dhawan, B.N. (1991): Methods for biological assessment of plant medicines. In: R.O.B. Wijesekera (Ed.), *The Medicinal Plant Industry*, 77–84. Boca Raton, Fla.: CRC Press.

Dhawan, B.N. (1995): Research priorities in natural products having CNS effects. *Curr. Sci.* **68**, 202–204.

Dhawan, B.N., Rastogi, R.P. (1991): Recent developments from Indian medicinal plants. In: R.O.B. Wijesekera (Ed.), *The Medicinal Plant Industry*, 185–208. Boca Raton, CRC Press.

Dixit, V.K., Varma, K.C. (1976): Effect of essential oil of leaves of *Blumea lacera* on central nervous system. *Ind. J. Pharmacol.* **8**, 7–11.

Dixit, V.K., Varma, K.C. (1979): Effect of essential oil of rhizomes of *Hedychium coronarium* and *Hedychium spicatum* on the central nervous system. *Ind. J. Pharmacol.* **11**, 147–149.

Dubey, M.P., Srimal, R.C., Patnaik, G.K., Dhawan, B.N. (1974): Hypotensive and spasmolytic activities of coleonol, active constituent of *Coleus forshkohlii. Briq. Ind. J. Pharmacol.* **6**, 15.

Dutta, S.C., Bhattacharya, S.K., Ray, A.B. (1976): Flower alkaloids of Alstonia scholaris. *Planta Med.* **30**, 86–89.

Ghosh, D., Anand Kumar, A. (1983): Anti-inflammatory and analgesic activities of Gangetin—a pterocarpinoid from *Desmodium pulchellum*. *Ind. J. Pharmacol.* **15**, 391–402.

Ghosh, D., Thejomoorthy, P., Veluchamy (1983): Anti-inflammatory and analgesic activities of oleoanolic acid 3-5-glucoside (RDG-1) from *Randia dumetorium* (Rubiaceae). *Ind. J. Pharmacol.* **15**, 331–342.

Ghosal, S., Dutta, G.K., Bhattacharya, S.K. (1972): Erythrina-chemical and pharmacological evaluation. II: Alkaloids of *Erythrina variegata L. J. Pharmaceut. Sci.* **61**, 1274–1277.

Ghosal, S. Sharma, P. V., Chaudhari, R. K. (1974): Chemical Constituents of Gentianaceae X: Xanthone-*o*-glucosides of *Swertia purpurascens* Wall.*J. Pharmaceut. Sci.* **63**, 1286–1290.

Gopalkrishnan, C., Shankaranarayan, D., Kameswaran, L., Natarajan, S. (1979):

Pharmacological investigations of tylophorine, the major alkaloid of *Tylophora indica*. *Ind. J. Med. Res.* **69**, 513-520.

Gopalkrishnan, C., Shankaranarayanan, D., Nazimuddin, S.K., et al. (1980): Anti-inflammatory and CNS depressant activities of *Calophyllium inophyllum* and *Mesua ferrea*. *Ind. J. Pharmacol.* **12**, 181-191.

Hylands, P.J., Nisbet, L.J. (1991): The search for molecular diversity (1): Natural products. *Ann. Rep. Med. Chem.* **26**, 259-270.

Jamwal, K.S., Anand, K.K., Chopra, I.C. (1962): Pharmacological properties of a crystalline substance (osthol) isolated from *Prangos pabularia* Ludl. *Arch. Int. Pharmacodyn.* **138**, 400-411.

Kar, K., Mukherji, K.C., Dhawan, B.N. (1977): Characterisation of neuromuscular blocking property of isococculidine. *Ind. J. Exp. Biol.* **15**, 547-551.

Karanth, K.S., Haridas, K.K., Gunasundari, S., Guruswami, M.N. (1980): Effect of *Celastrus paniculatus* on learning process. *Arogya—J. Health Sci.* **6**, 137-139.

Karanth, K.S., Padma, T.K., Guruswami, M.N. (1981): Influence of celastrus oil on learning and memory. *Arogya—J. Health Sci.* **7**, 83-84.

Kulkarni, S.K., Verma, A. (1992): Prevention of development of tolerance and dependence to opiate in mice by BR-16A (Mentat R), a herbal psychotropic preparation. *Ind. J. Exp. Biol.* **30**, 885-888.

Kumar, A., Pandey, V.B., Seth, K.K., et al. (1986): Pharmacological actions of fumariline isolated from *Fumaria indica* seeds. *Planta Med.* **52**, 323-325.

Lahon, L.C., Khanikor, H.N., Ahmad, N. (1979): Preliminary study of local anaesthetic activity of *Euphorbia nerifolia Linn. Ind. J. Pharmacol.* **11**, 239-240.

Madan, B.R., Khanna, N.K., Mahatma, G.P., et al. (1974): Further studies on some pharmacological actions of gindarine hydrochloride—an alkaloid of *Stephania glabra* (Roxb) Miers. *Ind. J. Pharmacol.* **6**, 97-102.

Mahatma, O.P., Rathore, O.S., Pancholi, M.S. (1987): Further studies on some pharmacological action of gindarinine hydrochloride—an alkaloid of *Stephania glabra* (Roxb) Miers. *Ind. Drugs* **24**, 537-541.

Mishra, P.K., Agarwal, R.K. (1988): Some pharmacological actions of the essential oil of *Luvunga scandens. Fitoterap.* **59**, 441-448.

Mukherjee, K.C., Patnaik, G.K., Bhakuni, D.S., Dhawan, B.N. (1984): Mechanism of neuromuscular blocking action of isocorydine methochloride : A new quaternary alkaloid from *Cocculus laurifolius* DC. *Ind. J. Exp. Biol.* **22**, 54-56.

Nazimuddin, S.K., Viswanathan, S., Kulanthaivel, P., et al. (1980): Pharmacological studies on the alkaloid fraction of *Stephania wightii* Dunn. *Ind. J. Med. Res.* **71**, 476-479.

Palanicherry, S., Nagarajan, S. (1990): Analgesic activity of *Cassia alata* leaf extract and Kaempferol 3-0-sophoroside. *J. Ethnopharmacol.* **29**, 73-78.

Patnaik. G.K., Dhawan, B.N. (1995): Pharmacology of medicinal plants. In: P. K. Seth, B.N. Dhawan (Eds.), *Current Research in Pharmacology in India* (1982-1987) 81-119. New Delhi: Indian National Science Academy.

Pradhan. S.N., De, N.N. (1953): Hayatin methiodide: A new curariform drug. *Br. J. Pharmacol.* **8**, 399-405.

Pradhan, S.N., Pandey, K., Badola, R.P. (1964): A clinical trial of hayatin methoiodide as a relaxant in 100 cases. *Br. J. Anaesth.* **10**, 604-611.

Rapaka, R.S., Makriyannis, A. (Ed.) (1987): Structure Activity Relationship of *the Cannabinoids*. Rockville, Md.: National Institute on Drug Abuse.

Rastogi, R.P., Dhawan, B.N., Dhar, M.M. (1987): Medicinal Plants. In: N.R. Rajgopal (Ed.), *40 Years of Research—A CSIR Overview*. 329-346. New Delhi: Council of Scientific and Industrial Research.

Rastogi, R.P., Mehrotra, B.N. (1990): *Compendium of Indian Medicinal Plants*, Vol. 1. New Delhi: CSIR Publication and Information Directorate.

Rastogi, R.P., Mehrotra, B.N. (1991): *Compendium of Indian Medicinal Plants*. Vol. 2. New Delhi: CSIR Publication and Information Directorate.

Rastogi, R.P., Mehrotra, B.N. (1993): *Compendium of Indian Medicinal Plants*, Vol. 3, 615-616. New Delhi: CSIR Publication and Information Directorate.

Sahai, R., Agarwal, S.K., Rastogi, R.P. (1980): Auriculoside—a new flavan glycoside from *Acacia auriculoformis*. *Phytochem* **19**, 1560-1562.

Sahu, N.C., Das. B.N. (1975): Local anaesthetic effect of the leaves of *Zizyphus jujuba*. *J. Res. Ind. Med*. **10**, 29-33.

Satyavati, G.V. (1984): Pharmacology of medicinal plants and other natural products. In: P.K. Das, B.N. Dhawan (Eds.), *Current Research in Pharmacology in India* (1975-1982), 119-146. New Delhi: Indian National Science Academy.

Seamon, K.B., Padgett. W., Daly, I.W. (1981): Forskolin: Unique diterpene activation of adenylate cyclase in membranes and in intact cells. *Proc. Nat. Acad. Sci. USA* **78**, 3363-3367.

Sen, A.K., Mahato, S.B., Dutta, N.L. (1975): Conyzic acid, a new diterpene resin acid from *Conyza stricta*. *Ind. J. Chem*. **13**, 504-507.

Seth, G., Kokate, C.K., Varma, K.C. (1976): Effect of essential oil of *Cymopogon citratus* on central nervous system. *Ind. J. Exp. Biol*. **14**. 370-374.

Sheth, U.K., Vaz, A., Deliwala, C.V., Bellare, R.A. (1963): Behavioural and pharmacological studies of a tranquillising fraction from the oil of *Celastrus paniculatus* (Malkanguni oil). *Arch. Int. Pharmacodyn*. **144**, 34-50.

Singh, G.B., Singh, S., Bani, S., et al. (1992): Anti-inflammatory activity of oleanolic acid in rat and mice. *J. Pharm. Pharmacol*. **44**, 456-458.

Singh, H., Kapoor, V.K. (1980): Investigation of Strychnos species: VI. Pharmacological studies of alkaloids of *Strychnos potatorum* seeds. *Planta Med*. **38**, 133-137.

Singh, H.K., Dhawan, B.N. (1982): Effect of *Bacopa monniera* Linn. (Brahmi) extract on avoidance response in rat. *J. Ethnopharmacol*. 5, 203-214.

Singh, H.K., Dhawan. B.N. (1994): Improvement of learning and memory by saponins of *Bacopa monniera*. *Canad. J. Physiol. Pharmacol*. **72**, S1, 407.

Singh, H.K., Rastogi, R.P., Srimal, R.C., Dhawan, B.N. (1988): Effect of Bacosides A and B on avoidance response in rats. *Phytotherap. Res*. **2**, 70-75.

Singh, H.K., Srimal, R.C., Dhawan, B.N. (1990): Neuropharmacologioal investigation on bacosides from *Bacopa monniera*. Actes du First Colloq. Europ. Ethnopharmacol. 319-321.

Singh, S., Garg, H.S., Khanna, N.M. (1976): Dysobinin, a new tetranortriterpene from *Dysoxylum binectariferum*. *Ind. J. Chem*. **14B**, 874-875.

Srivastava, A.K., Srivastava, B., Dixit, V. (1981): Pharmacological studies on fruits of *Melia azedarach* L. *J. Res. Ayur. Siddha* **2**, 200-263.

Tandon, S., Rastogi, R.P. (1979): Strictic acid—a novel deterpene from *Conyza stricta. Phytochem.* **18**, 494-495.

Viswanathan, S., Sambandam, P., Ramaswamy, S., Kameswaran, L. (1985): Studies on possible tolerance and mechanism of gossypin analgesia. *Ind. J. Exp. Biol.* **23**, 525-526.

Vohora, S.B.. Shamsi, M.A., Khan, M.S.Y. (1981): Antipyretic and analgesic studies on the diacetate of a new triterpenic acid isolated from *Corchorus depressus. J. Ethopharmacol.* **4**, 225-228.

7

Ginkgo Preparations: Biochemical, Pharmaceutical, and Medical Perspectives*

Otto Sticher

Phytomedicines that contain extracts from the leaves of Ginkgo biloba *have been used in Germany and France for a fairly long time to treat peripheral vascular disease and disturbances of cerebral function. In Europe, commercially available preparations based on the flavonoid and terpene lactone enriched dry extracts EGb 761 and LI 1370 have annual sales of about $500 million U.S.*

This chapter describes the chemistry, pharmacology, and clinical applications, as well as quality control, of G biloba and the phytomedicines that contain leaf extracts of this plant. Research conducted in our laboratory dealing with quality control is discussed in detail.

INTRODUCTION

Modern ginkgo phytomedicines are not derived from traditional medicine, although therapy with preparations of ginkgo can be traced back to the origins of Chinese herbal medicine. Extracts of *Ginkgo biloba* leaves were introduced into medical practice in 1965 as a result of the research of the firm of Dr. W. Schwabe, Karlsruhe, Germany. Today, preparations containing ginkgo leaf extracts are among the best selling phytopharmaceuticals in Europe, particularly

*Presented at the symposium on New Drug Development from Herbal Medicines in Neuropsychopharmacology, of the 19th CINP Congress, June 27-July 1, 1994, Washington, D.C.

Acknowledgments : The author wishes to thank everyone involved in this work, especially A. Hasler, a Ph.D. student in the group from 1986 to 1990. All the experimental work concerning the isolation and determination of flavonoids is described in detail in his thesis (Hasler, 1990). Dr. B. Meier, supervisor of this thesis, contributed many ideas to the work. Dr. Hasler's research was supported by a grant from Zeller Söhne AG, Romanshorn, Switzerland.

in France and Germany. The European ginkgo market, which seems to be increasing, sees annual sales of about $500 million U.S. This is not surprising in view of a population that encompasses more and more elderly people. The indications for ginkgo extracts are primarily for diseases that appear with advancing age.

CONSTITUENTS OF *GINKGO* LEAVES

Among the large number of polar and nonpolar compounds that have been isolated from ginkgo leaves are long-chain hydrocarbons and derivatives, alicy-

TABLE 1

Constituents of the leaves from *G biloba*

- *Terpenes*
 Diterpenes: ginkgolides A, B, C. J, M
 Sesquiterpene: bilobalide
 Polyprenols
 Steroids

- *Flavonoids*
 Flavone and flavonol glycosides
 Acylated flavonol glycosides
 Biflavonoids
 Flavane-3-ols
 Proanthocyanidins

- *Long-chain hydrocarbons and derivatives*
 Hydrocarbons
 Alcohols
 Aldehydes
 Ketones
 Acids

- *Alicyclic acids, cyclic compounds, carbohydrates, and derivatives*
 Shikimic acid, quinic acid, ascorbic acid, anacardiac acids (ginkgolic acid, hydroxyginkgolic acid), pinitol, sequoyitol, saccharose, high molecular polysaccharides

- Various compounds, such as (Z,Z)-4,4'-(1,4-pentadiene-1,5-diyl)diphenol, 6-hydroxykynuric acid, cytokinins, β-lectins, carotenodis

---

clic acids, cyclic compounds, carbohydrates and derivatives, flavonoids, isoprenoids (sterols, terpenoids), *(Z,Z)*-4,4'-(1,4-pentadiene-1,5-diyl)diphenol, 6-hydroxykynurenic acid, cytokinins, β-lectins, and carotenoids, among others (Table 1). The ginkgo extracts contain flavonoids and terpene lactones (ginkgolides and bilobalide) as active compounds. They affect vascular and cerebral metabolic processes and inhibit platelet activating factor (PAF) (for recent reviews, see Sticher et al., 1991; Hölzl, 1992; Sticher, 1993a, 1993b; and references cited therein).

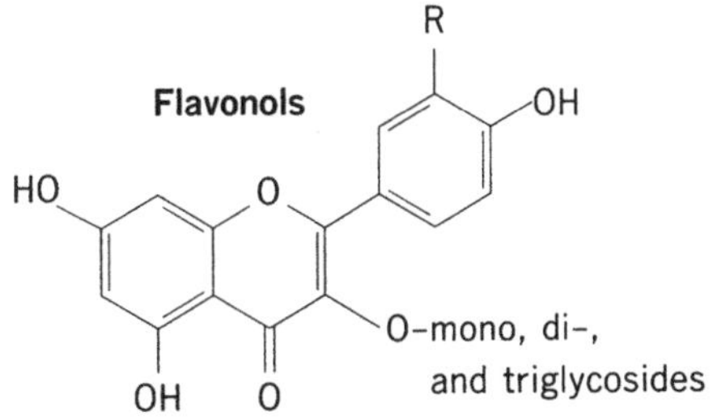

R	
H	kaempferol derivative
OH	quercetin derivative
OCH$_3$	isorhamnetin derivative

R$_1$	
H	kaempferol derivative
OH	quercetin derivative
R$_2$	H or glucose
R$_3$	H or glucose

Coumaric acid ester of flavonols

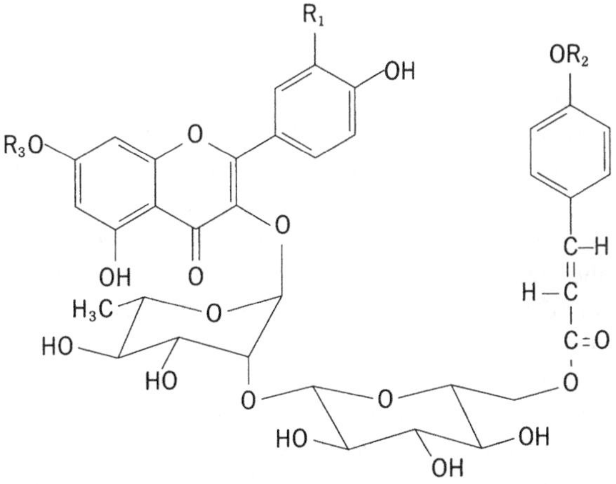

Figure 1. Examples of flavonoid glycoside structures isolated from leaves of *G biloba*.

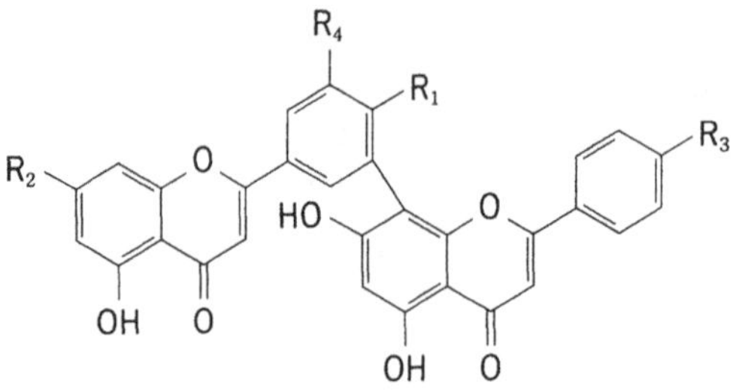

R_1	R_2	R_3	R_4	
OH	OH	OH	H	Amentoflavone
OCH_3	OH	OH	H	Bilobetin
OCH_3	OCH_3	OH	H	Ginkgetin
OCH_3	OH	OCH_3	H	Isoginkgetin
COH_3	OCH_3	OCH_3	H	Sciadopitysin
OCH_3	OH	OH	OCH_3	5′-Methoxybilobetin

Figure 2. Biflavones isolated from leaves of *G biloba*.

The main known flavonoids of ginkgo leaves (Fig. 1) represent a great variety of flavonol glycosides based on kaempferol and quercetin and occur as mono-, di-, and triglycosides. Minor flavonoid compounds are derived from isorhamnetin, myricetin, 3'-methyl myricetin (with a flavonol structure), as well as from apigenin and luteolin (with a flavone structure). Structurally interesting compounds include the flavonoid glycoside esters with coumaric acid. These acylated flavonol glycosides are useful lead compounds in the quality control of ginkgo preparations. In addition, nonglycosidic biflavonoids (Fig. 2), catechins, and proanthocyanidins have been isolated. The flavonoid substances, particularly the flavonol glycosides and the proanthocyanidins, could be partly responsible for the free radical scavenging activity of ginkgo extracts, which might play a significant role in their therapeutic actions (DeFeudis, 1991, and references cited therein).

The terpenoids (Fig. 3) are characteristic constituents of ginkgo and have either a diterpenoid structure, as with the five known ginkgolides, or a sesquiterpenoid structure in the case of bilobalide. These substances possess three lactone functions and a tertiary-butyl group, a combination that is unique in the plant kingdom. The structure of bilobalide shows a relationship to those of the ginkgolides. Biogenetically, bilobalide is a degradation product of the ginkgolides. Recent studies have indicated that the ginkgolides possess PAF antago-

R₁	R₂	R₃	Ginkgolide
OH	H	H	A
OH	OH	H	B
OH	OH	OH	C
OH	H	OH	J
H	OH	OH	M

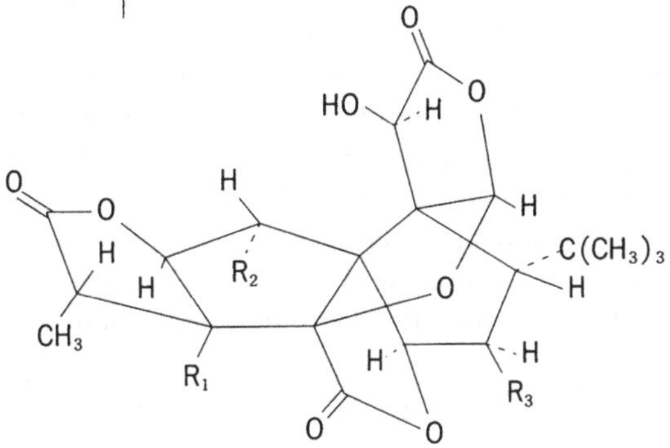

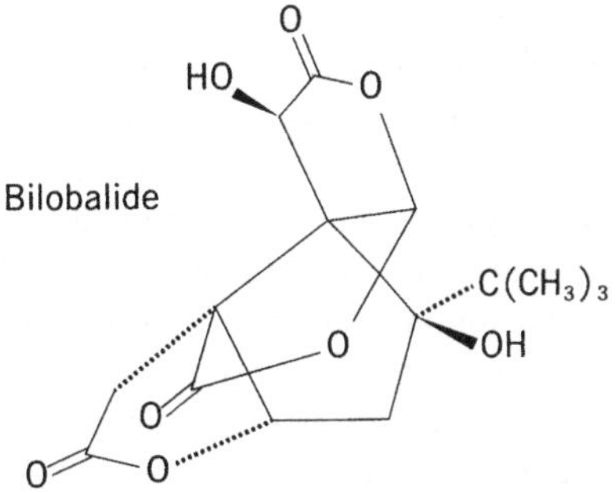

Bilobalide

Figure 3. Terpene lactones (ginkgolides and bilobalide) isolated from leaves of *G biloba*.

nist activity (DeFeudis, 1991, and references cited therein), while bilobalide has neuroprotective properties (Krieglstein, 1994).

PHARMACOLOGIC STUDIES

Pharmacologic studies have been performed mainly with extract EGb 761 (Schwabe, Karlsruhe) (see standard books, such as Fünfgeld, 1988; Braquet, 1988/1989; DeFeudis, 1991) and recently with LI 1370 (Lichtwer Pharma,

Berlin) (Hartmann & Schulz, 1991). These extracts are used to treat peripheral vascular disease and, more important, cerebral insufficiency (for recent reviews, see Hasler, 1990; Oberpichler-Schwenk & Krieglstein, 1992; Kleijnen & Knipschild, 1992a, 1992b; Krieglstein, 1994; and references cited therein).

Increased Blood Supply

The effects on blood vessels (vasorelaxation) and on blood flow (reduction of total-blood viscosity) may explain the increase in blood supply. Various mechanisms of action have been discussed with regard to vasorelaxation. Among these, the effects on prostaglandin metabolism, where there is increased synthesis of the vasodilating prostacyclin, and the radical scavenging properties of the extract are involved. The reduction of pathologically elevated total-blood viscosity seems to be due to a reduction in erythrocyte aggregation. Once again, the effects on prostaglandin metabolism, as well as the PAF antagonism of the extract, play roles in its action on blood flow and on other smooth-muscle organs.

Effects on Cerebral Function

Among other factors, increased tolerance to hypoxia, effects on energy metabolism, protection against ischemia, and antiedematous effects have been studied to demonstrate the effects of ginkgo extracts on experimentally damaged brain. Additionally, the extracts' actions regarding learning and memory, as well as its effects on neurotransmitter systems, have been studied.

The survival time of mice and rats exposed to lethal hypoxia have been markedly prolonged by the administration of ginkgo extract (Fig. 4). Similarly, the decline in brain energy metabolism and the onset of respiratory arrest in the hypoxic rat were delayed by ginkgo extract. The cerebroprotective substance responsible for these actions appears to be the nonflavonoid fraction that contains the ginkgolides and bilobalide.

In cerebral ischemia, the cerebroprotective effects found after administering ginkgo extract differ, depending on the ischemia model used. Statistically significant cerebral protection has been demonstrated with individual terpene lactones. Ginkgolides attenuate the neurotoxic effect of glutamate, which is released during ischemia and leads to a disruption of stimulated neurons. It seems likely that the effect of glutamate also enhances the production of PAF, which in turn can have a lethal effect on neurons. The neuroprotective effect therefore may be attributed to the PAF-antagonistic action of the ginkgolides. However, bilobalide exhibits the greatest cerebroprotective effect, and this terpene lactone shows no PAF-antagonistic activity. Its mechanism of action is still unclear.

The effects on learning capacity and memory are of interest in view of the

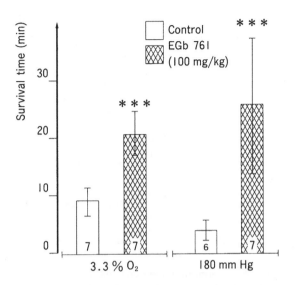

Figure 4. Increase in survival time of rats treated with EGb 761 under lethal hypoxia (Oberpichler–Schwenk & Krieglstein, 1992).

therapeutic use of ginkgo extracts in cerebral insufficiency. The results of studies performed thus far differ, depending on the age of the laboratory animals used. It appears that the extract has no effect on the learning behavior of young rats (eight months old), but improves learning in older animals (24 months old). The results of studies involving the cerebral noradrenergic system have also been variable. It has been demonstrated that ginkgo extract can abolish the age-related decline of the number of muscarinic receptors in the rat hippocampus. The normalization of age-related receptor deficits may represent a common mechanism of nootropics (drugs that stimulate cerebral metabolism).

From the foregoing discussion, it becomes clear that the pharmacologic actions of ginkgo extract are based on the radical scavenging properties and PAF antagonism of specific constituents, as well as unknown mechanisms.

Radical Scavenging Properties

The effects of ginkgo extract on vascular tone and blood coagulation, and its protective actions under ischemic conditions, can be partially explained by its radical scavenging properties. Various in vitro studies suggest that the flavonoid glycosides are responsible for these effects. However, flavonoid glycosides are relatively polar molecules and thus should not reach the brain. Therefore, other

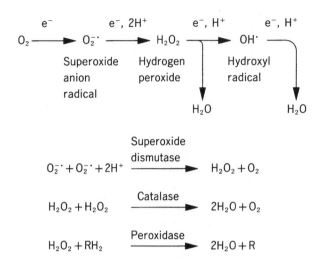

Figure 5. Formation and enzymatic inactivation of oxygen radicals (Oberpichler-Schwenk & Krieglstein, 1992).

substances or flavonoid metabolites must be considered with regard to radical scavenging properties at the neuronal level. Further studies are needed to clarify this question.

Free radicals are continuously formed within living tissues because of the incomplete reduction of oxygen (Fig. 5). Under normal conditions, specific enzymes prevent radical-induced tissue damage. Enhanced radical formation that occurs during ischemia and hypoxia may exceed the capacity of the enzymatic inactivation mechanisms. Oxygen radicals have a toxic effect on various enzyme systems, cell membranes, and cell functions (Fig. 6). Their action on membrane lipids could affect cell membrane permeability and thus promote the development of edema.

The interactions of eicosanoids (prostaglandins, thromboxane, prostacyclin, and leukotrienes) are of decisive relevance to vascular physiology. The dynamic equilibrium between prostacyclin and thromboxane A_2 plays an essential role in the pathogenesis of various circulatory disorders. Prostacyclin is responsible for vasodilation and the inhibition of platelet aggregation, while thromboxane A_2 causes vasoconstriction and enhanced platelet aggregation. The appropriate equilibrium can be adversely affected by lipid peroxides. Lipid peroxides are formed by free radicals, particularly in the reoxygenation phase after ischemia, and inhibit prostacyclin synthetase, which can lead to a relative excess of thromboxane A_2.

Another site of action involves the adenyl cyclase-phosphodiesterase system,

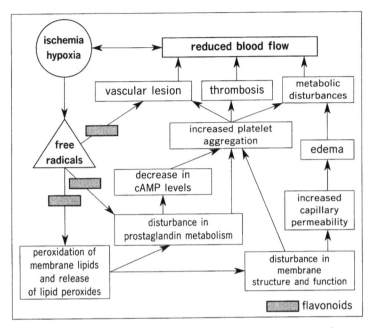

Figure 6. Free radical scavenging activity of flavonoids from *G biloba* (modified according to Chatterjee, 1984).

which regulates intracellular cyclic adenosine monophosphate (cAMP) levels. Adenyl cyclase is inhibited by an excess of thromboxane A_2, and this leads to a decrease in cAMP levels. High cAMP levels promote platelet stability, whereas low levels promote platelet aggregation. Ginkgo extract also protects erythrocytes against hemolysis and reduces capillary permeability via membrane stabilization, which could prevent the formation of edema.

PAF Antagonism

The constituents of ginkgo extract with PAF-antagonistic activity are the ginkgolides. In particular, ginkgolide B has been found to be a very active PAF antagonist. PAF represents an ether-phospholipid (Fig. 7), which is formed and released by leukocytes, macrophages, thrombocytes, and endothelial cells in response to specific stimuli (Fig. 8). It possesses the property of triggering platelet aggregation, and is also involved in inflammatory reactions, the elevation of vascular permeability, and the contraction of smooth muscles. For example, macrophages, leukocytes, and thrombocytes respond to antigen binding with release of this physiologically active phospholipid. PAF then binds to PAF

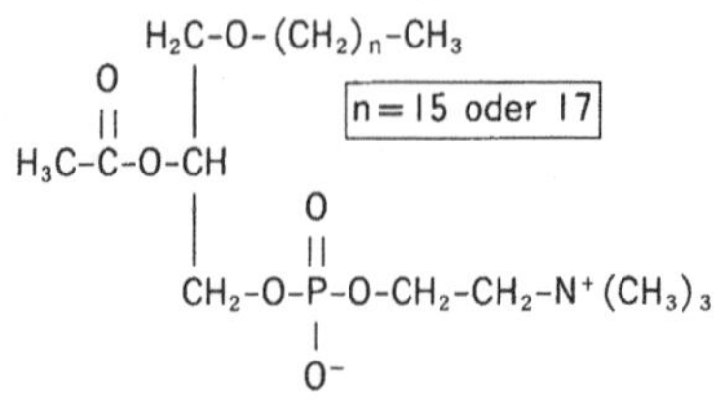

$$H_2C-O-(CH_2)_n-CH_3$$

$$\begin{array}{c} O \\ \parallel \\ H_3C-C-O-CH \end{array} \quad \boxed{n = 15 \text{ oder } 17}$$

$$\begin{array}{c} O \\ \parallel \\ CH_2-O-P-O-CH_2-CH_2-N^+(CH_3)_3 \\ \mid \\ O^- \end{array}$$

Figure 7. Structural formula of the platelet-activating factor (PAF).

receptors on target cells (e.g., vascular endothelial cells, leukocytes, mast cells, platelets), which leads to the release of mediators (including histamine and eicosanoids) and various physiologic reactions, such as vasodilation and platelet aggegation. These actions are responsible for asthma, inflammation, and anaphylaxis. PAF antagonists block the PAF receptors of target cells. The inhibition of platelet aggregation appears to be the most relevant action associated with ginkgo use. PAF receptors have been detected in the brain, and thus there is a possible relation with the protective action of ginkgo extract against oxygen deficits in the brain. This is a logical conclusion since PAF causes various reactions similar to those occurring in hypoxic tissues.

CLINICAL APPLICATIONS

Pharmacologic research on ginkgo extracts EGb 761 and LI 1370 has led to the main areas of application described in the following (for recent reviews, see Hasler, 1990; Kleijnen and Knipschild, 1992a, 1992b; & references cited therein).

Cerebral Insufficiency

The main indication for the use of ginkgo extract is for the treatment of cerebral insufficiency. Among the disorders affecting the elderly that would be typical of cerebral insufficiency and are claimed to be relieved by treatment with ginkgo extract are difficulties with concentration and memory, absentmindedness, confusion, lack of energy, tiredness, decreased physical performance, depressed mood, and anxiety. These symptoms have been associated with impaired cerebral circulation, and sometimes they are thought to be early indications of dementia of either the degenerative or multiple infarct type, but often no explanation can be found (Kleijnen and Knipschild, 1992a, 1992b). Headache, vertigo, and tinnitus are frequent complaints with cerebral insufficiency.

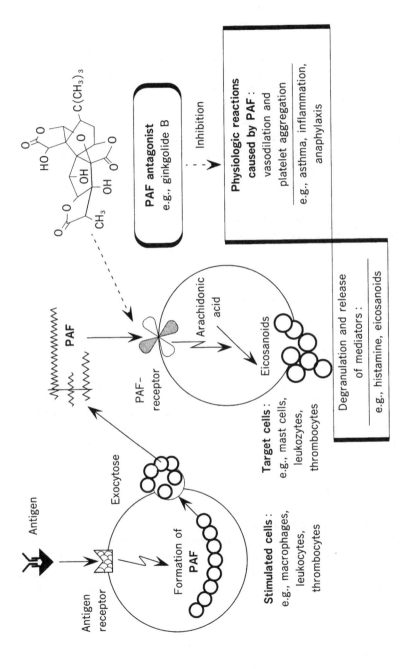

Figure 8. Formation and pharmacologic effects of PAF (modified according to Weber, 1986).

These deteriorations in mental functions can be arrested or slowed by proper training. Various studies with suitable test methods have shown that ginkgo extract improves the results. Long-term treatment with ginkgo extract significantly improved pathologically altered electroencephalograph (EEG) findings in patients with cerebral insufficiency. This was accompanied by an attenuation of major symptoms, such as headache and vertigo.

According to Kleijnen and Knipschild (1992a, 1992b), 40 controlled trials on cerebral insufficiency have been published, eight of which are of good quality. The others have shortcomings as to methodology, including small numbers of patients; inadequate descriptions of randomization, patient characteristics, and effect measurements; and poor presentation of data. Although a positive effect of ginkgo as compared with placebo in patients with cerebro-organic syndromes could be demonstrated in most of the trials, the therapeutic benefit of nootropics is disputed. It thus is not surprising that the use of ginkgo extract to treat dementia syndromes is not unanimously accepted.

Peripheral Blood Flow Disorders

Many experimental and clinical studies support the efficacy of ginkgo extract in peripheral blood flow disorders. The most common causes of occlusive arterial disease are based on artherosclerotic modification of the vascular wall. Obliterative artherosclerosis is a disease of the intima, characterized by hardening of the wall, loss of elasticity, and narrowing of the lumen. It is a polyethiologic disease promoted by various factors, particularly hypertension, hyperlipemia, smoking, lack of exercise, and diabetes mellitus. The initial signs are arterial circulatory disorders of the limbs. The severity of the arterial perfusion insufficiency is classified in four stages, called Fontaine's stages. The value of ginkgo extract in stage II has been repeatedly proved by a significant increase in the distance the patient can walk pain-free. A prophylactic action can be expected in stage I.

Dizziness, Hearing Disorders, Tinnitus

Vertigo, hearing disorders, and tinnitus may have many and varied causes, but they are often associated with insufficient perfusion in the brain or inner ear. Vertigo is regarded as one of the pathologic conditions that respond best to ginkgo extract. This, and its variously established efficacy in tinnitus and deteriorated hearing performance, have contributed to the increased use of ginkgo extract.

QUANTITATION OF FLAVONOIDS
AND TERPENE LACTONES

The demonstrated importance of the ginkgo market would suggest theoretically that there have been a large number of publications in the fieid of quality control. However, the opposite is true. There are far more papers on most of the various drugs listed in pharmacopoeias, even if their importance is limited. To date, there are no published general quality standards for ginkgo leaves and the ginkgo phytomedicines, although laboratories in various universities are actively involved in the analysis of ginkgo constituents. It appears that the marketing strategies of most companies that produce ginkgo preparations do not permit the publication of company-developed quality control standards.

The fact that no pharmacopoeial monograph entitled "Ginkgo Folium" exists is indicative of the fact that no official standards have yet been established. The standardization of phytomedicines serves primarily as a precaution as to the quality of medicinal plant extracts. The most favored objects for standardization are the active compounds, which, in the case of ginkgo leaves, are the flavonoids and terpene lactones. In this regard, our primary aim was the development of a suitable method for quality control of the flavonoid glycosides that occur in ginkgo (for recent reviews, see Sticher, 1992, 1993a, 1993b).

Qualitative and Quantitative Determination of Flavonoids

Hydrolysis of the glycosides, followed by a spectrophotometric determination of the aglycones as an aluminum chelate complex, is the method currently used to determine the concentration levels of flavonoids in herbal drugs. This method, described in several pharmacopoeias, is not very specific and permits only an approximate estimation of the total flavonoids in plants. In the case of ginkgo leaves, this method is not reproducible owing to an incomplete extraction of the polar flavonol glycosides (acetone extraction), and probably to the large amount of interfering proanthocyanidins. Further, a detailed determination of the qualitative and quantitative composition of the aglycones is not possible (Hasler, 1990; Sticher, 1993a, 1993b). On the other hand, reversed-phase high-performance liquid chromatography (RP-HPLC) and subsequent diode-array detection allows for a selective analysis of the ginkgo flavonoids.

There have been only a few investigations on the separation and quantitative determination of ginkgo flavonoids. Briançon-Scheid and co-workers (1982, 1983), Song (1986), Pietta et al. (1988), and Schennen (1988) reported HPLC separations of biflavones. According to present knowledge, the biflavones represent characteristic markers for the identification of ginkgo leaves, but they do not show the desired activities and so are not suitable for use as standards (for details, see Sticher, 1993b).

Determination of the Aglycones After Hydrolysis

A direct determination of the naturally occurring flavonoid glycosides that belong to the active principles of ginkgo extracts would be desirable. In the case of ginkgo, this is not possible because the flavonoid profile is very complex, and so analysis during pharmaceutical quality control would be rather tedious. Additionally, most of the reference compounds are not commercially available. On the other hand, the great variety of flavonoid glycosides can be reduced by hydrolysis to the three major aglycones of kaempferol, quercetin, and isorhamnetin (Fig. 9). As a result, a simple, rapid, and reproducible method for the standardization of ginkgo extracts has been realized (Hasler, 1990; Hasler et al., 1990a, 1990b). The workup procedure consists of two basic steps: extraction and hydrolysis of the glycosides, and sample cleanup. Extraction and hydrolysis are performed by refluxing the pulverized plant material or a plant extract with 10 ml hydrochloric acid (25%) in 70 ml methanol for 60 minutes. Sample cleanup is carried out using C_{18} solid-phase extraction cartridges. An aliquot of the final preparation is then subjected to HPLC. The flavonoid aglycones can be easily analyzed by RP-HPLC using a methanol-water gradient with 0.5% v/v ortho-phosphoric acid and ultraviolet (UV) detection at 370 nm. Similar methods have been described by Wagner et al. (1989) and by Schennen (1988). The reduction of the genuine glycosides by hydrolysis is an accepted method in the quality control of phytomedicines and has been described by our laboratory for the standardization of willow and hawthorn preparations (Meier et al., 1985: Rehwald et al., 1994).

The obtained aglycone content (Fig. 10) is finally converted to a ginkgo flavonol glycoside content. This is done in accordance with the practice in the pharmaceutical industry, although no published data are available. The producers of ginkgo preparations convert the obtained aglycone content into a "ginkgo flavone" glycoside content for marketing purposes. As ginkgo flavone glycosides, flavonol coumaroyl ester glycosides, with an average molecular weight of approximately 760, are documented. Thus, the final flavonoid content is once again higher. A standardization based on these acylated flavonol glycosides is acceptable from a pharmaceutical viewpoint because they are leading substances in ginkgo leaves and extracts.

A typical HPLC chromatogram of a hydrolyzed ginkgo extract is shown in Figure 11. Kaempferol and quercetin are the main peaks. The concentration of isorhamnetin is approximately five times lower than that of either of the main aglycones. The very small minor peaks represent additional aglycones, such as apigenin and luteolin. Our investigations have shown that dried ginkgo leaves

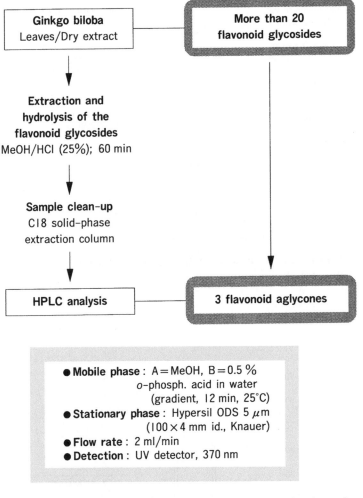

Figure 9. Workup procedure and HPLC determination of flavonoid aglycones from *G. biloba*.

obtained on the commercial market contain an aglycone content of 0.2-0.4% w/w, corresponding to a calculated ginkgo flavonol glycoside content of 0.5 to 1% w/w. Green leaves are considered to be of higher quality. However, with respect to the flavonoid content, no significant differences could be seen in our ontogenetic studies (with the exception of those during the month of May, when young leaves were analyzed) (Fig. 12).

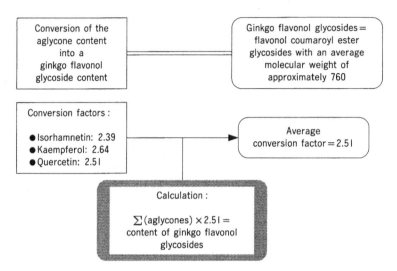

Figure 10. Conversion of the aglycone content into a ginkgo flavonol glycoside content.

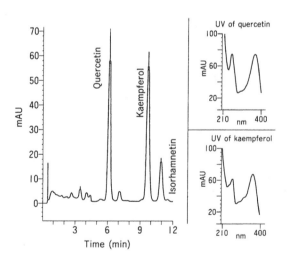

Figure 11. HPLC chromatogram of a ginkgo leaf extract after hydrolysis of the flavonoid glycosides.

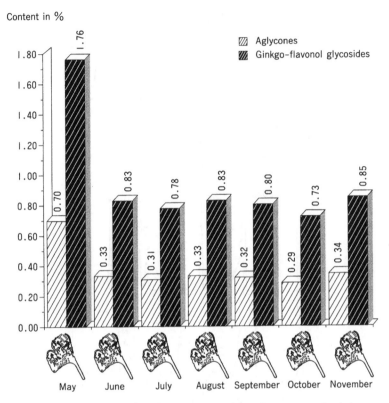

Content in %

Figure 12. Concentration of flavonoid aglycones and ginkgo flavonol glycosides depending on the harvest time (leaves of a female tree, Zürich, Mythenquai, calculated with reference to the dried leaves).

Determination of the Flavonoid Aglycones and Detection of the Biflavones

A second RP-HPLC method (MeOH-THF gradient with 0.5% orthophosphoric acid) allows, in addition to the quantitative determination of the flavonoid aglycones, a qualitative determination of the biflavones during a single run (Fig. 13) (for details, see Hasler, 1990; Hasler et al., 1992). This analytical method ensures that authentic ginkgo leaves were used as the starting material for extraction. The ubiquitous aglycones alone are not specific enough to identify *G biloba* leaves or full ginkgo extracts. Also, this method cannot be applied to special extracts, such as EGb 761, where the biflavonoids have been removed.

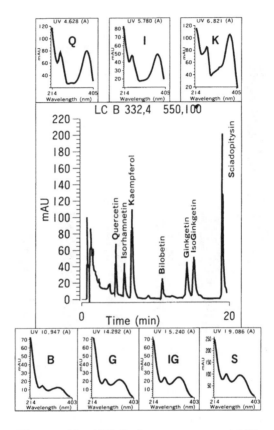

Figure 13. HPLC chromatogram and UV spectra of the aglycones and biflavones of a hydrolyzed ginkgo leaf extract.

Fingerprint Analysis of the Genuine Occurring Flavonoids

A third analytical method (isopropanol/THF [25:65]-acetonitrile gradient with 0.5% orthophosphoric acid) gives a fingerprint analysis of all naturally occurring ginkgo flavonoids during one 30-minute HPLC run (Fig. 14) (for details, see Hasler, 1990; Hasler et al., 1992). With this method, it is possible to identify unambiguously 22 flavonoid glycosides, six flavonoid aglycones, and five biflavones in leaves and extracts from the elution order and UV spectra. Because of the complex mixture of very polar (triglycosides), polar (mono- and di-glycosides) and apolar flavonoids (biflavones), the separation requires a sophisticated HPLC instrument consisting of a three-pump system and a diode-array

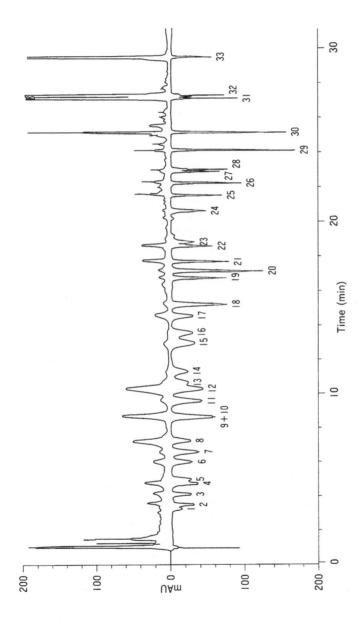

Figure 14. Fingerprint chromatogram of an ethanolic extract of *G biloba* (upper chromatogram) and of the isolated flavonoids and reference compounds (lower chromatogram).

detector. Fingerprint analysis is especially useful in performing stability tests. It can be shown that the flavonoid glycosides and the biflavones are stable, and that the ratios of these compounds do not change. An increase in the aglycones and a decrease in the glycosides indicate that an undesired degradation process has occurred in the extract. The fingerprint analysis allows for the identification of the very typical flavonol coumaroyl ester glycosides 21 [quercetin''3-O-rha(2''→ 1''')glc(6'''→ 1'''')coumaroyl ester] and 22 [kaempferol''3-O-rha(2''→ 1''')glc(6'''→ 1'''')coumaroyl ester]. Both are well separated from each other and from other compounds (Fig. 14 and Table 2).

A fingerprint HPLC separation of flavonoids from ginkgo leaves was also described by Wagner et al. (1989). In their study, 20 peaks were detected within 55 minutes, but only two flavonoids (rutin and astragalin), the four biflavones (bilobetin, ginkgetin/isoginkgetin, and sciadopitysin), ginkgol, shikimic acid, and 6-hydroxykynurenic acid could be identified. Pietta et al. (1991) reported an HPLC method for the separation of 15 known ginkgo flavonoids within 50 minutes. Using reference compounds, six flavonoids were identified. The other flavonoid glycosides were assigned by their UV spectra using a diode-array detector, although their absorptions were less than 10 milliabsorption units (mAU). Such assignments, without any supplementary data, are very speculative. In both papers (Wagner et al., 1989; Pietta et al., 1991), the separation and identification of the flavonoids are not well developed and are incomplete. Lobstein et al. (1991) used gradient elution with acetonitrile and 0.1 N phosphoric acid to separate flavonoids and biflavones within 50 minutes but with no diode-array detector coupled to the HPLC. Additionally, the lack of reference compounds prevented complete peak assignment. Only kaempferol- and quercetin-3-O-coumaroyl glucorhamnosides and the biflavones in leaves were quantitated.

Qualitative and Quantitative Determination of Terpene Lactones

Unfortunately, analysis of the terpene lactones was much more difficult to accomplish due to their low concentration in the leaves (according to Van Beek et al. [1991], very often below 0.1% w/w). Furthermore, these compounds show very poor UV absorption characteristics and first must be extracted from a highly complex matrix because no suitable sample cleanup method has yet been described. Between 1981 and 1993, several HPLC (Guth et al., 1981; Lobstein-Guth et al., 1983; Teng, 1988; Komoda et al., 1988; Pietta et al., 1990; Van Beek et al., 1991; Van Beek & Lelyveld, 1992; Pietta et al., 1992; Flesch et al., 1992), thin-layer chromatographic (TLC) (Wagner et al., 1989; Teng, 1988; Tallevi & Kurz, 1991; Van Beek & Lelyveld, 1993), gas chromatographic-mass spectrometric (GC-MS) (Carrier et al., 1991; Chauret et al., 1991), gas chromatographic (GC)

TABLE 2

The gradient elution profile of the naturally occurring flavonoids of *G biloba*

No.	t_R	Flavonoid
1	3.21	3-O-{2-O-[6-O-(p-Coumaroyl)-β-D-glucosyl]-α-L-rhamnosyl}-7-O-(β-D-glucosyl)quercetin
2	3.47	3-O-[2-O, 6-O-Bis(α-L-rhamnosyl)-β-D-glucosyl]quercetin
3	4.09	3-O-[2-O, 6-O-Bis(α-L-rhamnosyl)-β-D-glucosyl]isorhamnetin
4	4.71	3-O-[2-O, 6-O-Bis(α-L-rhamnosyl)β-D-glucosyl]kaempferol
5	4.97	3-O-[6-O-(α-L-Rhamnosyl)-β-D-glucosyl]myricetin
6	5.96	3-O-[6-O-(α-L-Rhamnosyl)-β-D-glucosyl]-3'-methylmyricetin
7	6.53	3-O-(2-O-{6-O-[p-(β-D-Glucosyl)coumaroyl]-β-D-glucosyl}-α-L-rhamnosyl)quercetin
8	7.19	3-O-[6-O-(α-L-Rhamnosyl)-β-D-glucosyl]quercetin
9	8.73	3-O-(2-O-{6-O-[p-(β-D-Glucosyl)coumaroyl]-β-D-glucosyl}-α-L-rhamnosyl)kaempferol
10	8.73	3-O-[6-O-(α-L-Rhamnosyl)-β-D-glucosyl]isorhamnetin
11	9.68	3-O-(β-D-Glucosyl)quercetin
12	10.37	3-O-[6-O-(α-L-Rhamnosyl)-β-D-glucosyl]kaempferol
13	10.74	3-O-[2-O-(β-D-Glucosyl)-α-L-rhamnosyl]quercetin
14	11.39	3-O-(β-D-Glucosyl)isorhamnetin
15	13.00	3-O-(β-D-Glucosyl)kaempferol
16	13.58	7-O-(β-D-Glucosyl)apigenin
17	14.58	3-O-[2-O-(β-D-Glucosyl)-α-L-rhamnosyl]kaempferol
18	15.22	3-O-(α-L-Rhamnosyl)quercetin
19	16.65	3'-O-(β-D-Glucosyl)luteolin
20	17.05	3-O-(α-L-Rhamnosyl)kaempferol
21	17.60	3-O-{2-O-[6-O-(p-Coumaroyl)-β-D-glucosyl]-α-L-rhamnosyl}quercetin
22	18.51	3-O-{2-O-[6-O-(p-Coumaroyl)-β-D-glucosyl]-α-L-rhamnosyl}kaempferol
23	18.76	Myricetin
24	20.60	Luteolin
25	21.50	Quercetin
26	22.22	Apigenin
27	22.76	Isorhamnetin
28	22.91	Kaempferol
29	24.02	Amentoflavon
30	25.06	Bilobetin
31	27.00	Ginkgetin
32	27.17	Isoginkgetin
33	29.35	Sciadopitysin

(Hasler & Meier, 1992; Huh and Staba, 1993), nuclear magnetic resonance imaging (NMR) (Van Beek et al., 1993), and biologic methods (Wagner & Steinke, 1991; Steinke et al., 1993) have been developed for the analysis of the terpene lactones in ginkgo leaves and extracts. Most of these methods either give unsatisfactory results, are inadequate or cannot be reproduced because of the lack of important experimental data, or are not suitable for routine analysis for the quality control of phytomedicines.

In the following, the HPLC method developed by Van Beek et al. (1991) and a recently presented GC method (Hasler & Meier, 1992) are discussed.

HPLC Determination of Terpene Lactones

The selective extraction of ginkgo leaves (van Beek et al., 1991) with methanol-water (10:90), or of phytomedicines with water, followed by sample cleanup with polyamide and C_{18} solid-phase extraction columns in series, gives extracts that can be readily analyzed by RP-HPLC with water-methanol (67:33) as the mobile phase and refractive index (RI) detection (Fig. 15). Boiling water with a low percentage of methanol has been found to be a selective primary extraction solvent for the ginkgolides. Although many interfering compounds are coextracted, they can be removed using the described sample cleanup procedure. The polyamide column removes most of the phenolics. The terpene lactones are retained on the C_{18} column by elution with a solvent of low methanol content. By increasing the methanol content, the terpene lactones can be removed from the column. This cleanup procedure allows for the analysis of the terpene lactones if RI detection is used rather than the usual UV detection.

All the leaves and phytomedicines investigated were found to contain bilobalide and ginkgolides, although large differences between different leaf batches or ginkgo preparations from different manufacturers were observed. The leaves investigated were from seven different sources. Leaves obtained from France contained the highest amounts of total terpene lactones, whereas all the others contained much less (Table 3). The total concentration of terpenoids was found to vary by a factor of 40. In all of the samples examined, the bilobalide content was equal to or higher than that of the total ginkgolides.

Van Beek et al. (1991) have shown that the controlled preparation of partially purified ginkgo phytomedicines, such as Tebonin, Rökan, and Tanakan, contain much higher concentrations of ginkgolides and bilobalide than do other, especially Dutch, preparations that are prepared according to the homeopathic pharmacopoeia (Table 3). The total concentration of terpenoids varied by a factor of 18. One French preparation (Ginkgogink) was completely different from all others. It contained high concentrations of all the ginkgolides, but bilobalide could not be detected. Since bilobalide is the major terpenoid in all of

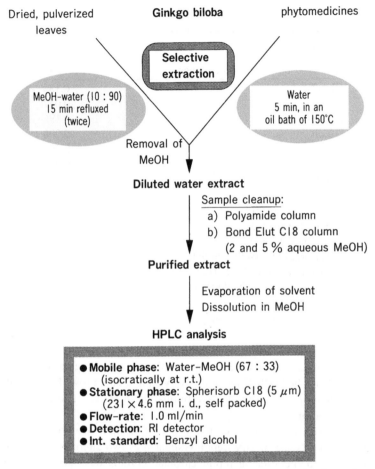

Figure 15. Workup procedure and HPLC determination of terpene lactones (bilobalide and ginkgolides) from *G biloba* according to Van Beek et al. (1991).

the leaves and other phytomedicines investigated, this finding suggested that it had been selectively removed during the manufacturing process. Additionally, the chromatogram of this preparation revealed extra peaks that were not present in any other sample of leaves or phytomedicines.

Although this method yields good results, the cleanup procedure is rather time consuming and depends heavily on the quality of commercially available C_{18} columns. Therefore, Pietta et al. (1992) presented a single-step purification procedure using Bakerbond alumina cartridges together with improved

TABLE 3

Ginkgolide and bilobalide concentrations in leaves and phytomedicines*

Leaves (origin) / phytomedicines	Content (%)
Chinese	0.134
Dutch	0.037
Dutch (1989)	0.196
Dutch	0.006
French	0.266
French	0.252
German	0.032
Tanakan (France)	0.220
Rökan (Germany)	0.192
Tebonin (Germany)	0.213
Geriaforce (The Netherlands)	0.017
Ginkgoplant (The Netherlands)	0.013
Naphyto DØ (The Netherlands)	0.012
Ginkgogink (France)	0.111

* From Van Beek et al. (1991).

chromatographic conditions using C_8 Nucleosil 300 (5 μm) and 1-propanol-THF-H_2O (1:13:86) with UV detection at 220 nm. According to these authors, this recently published HPLC method is very simple and allows for a rapid and clean determination of ginkgolides and bilobalide in extracts and their pharmaceutical preparations.

Note: After this review was written, evaporative light scattering (ELS) and thermospray-mass spectrometry were investigated as two alternative methods for the detection and quantitative liquid chromatographic determination of ginkgolides and bilobalide in leaf extracts and phytopharmaceuticals (Camponovo et al., 1995). The coupling of HPLC with an ELS detector seems to be particularly appropriate for routine analysis, whereas that of thermospray with mass spectrometry is not suitable owing to high price of this sophisticated apparatus and the limited accuracy of the quantitative results.

GC Determination of Terpene Lactones

It now seems that GC is the method of choice for the analysis of terpene lactones in ginkgo extracts. Hasler and Meier (1992) presented a well-validated and fast (20 minutes) capillary GC method that allows the determination of all terpene lactones after extraction, purification, and conversion to trimethylsilyl

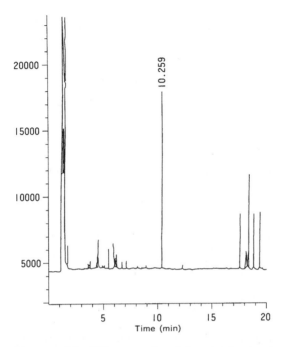

Figure 16. GC traces of a ginkgo total extract after the extraction, purification, and derivatization procedure according to Hasler and Meier (1992). Peak at t_R: 10.259 = trimethylsilyl ether of bilobalide; peaks at $t_R > 17$ minutes = trimethylsilyl ethers of the ginkgolides A, B, C, and J, and cholesterol as an internal standard (see Fig. 17).

derivatives (Figs. 16 and 17). Compared with RP-HPLC, capillary GC has the inherent advantage of much greater separation capacity and higher resolution. Additionally, the purification steps essential to HPLC analysis are not as critical when using capillary GC.

GINKGO EXTRACTS AND COMMERCIAL PRODUCTS

The extract as an Active Ingredient of Phytomedicines

In phytotherapy, the extract in its entirety is the active ingredient. There has been a gradual transition from the view that phytopharmaceuticals must contain all of the constituents of the initial herbal material in their natural proportions

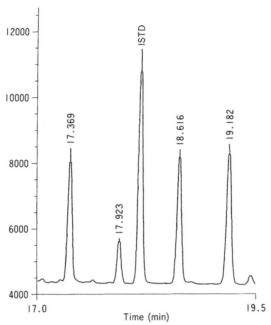

Figure 17. GC traces of the section between t_R 17.0 and 19.5 minutes of the chromatogram in Figure 16. The peaks show the trimethylsilyl derivatives of the ginkgolides. Ginkgolide A = peak at t_R: 17.369; ginkgolide B = peak at t_R: 18.616; ginkgolide C = peak at t_R: 19.182; ginkgolide J = peak at t_R: 17.923; ISTD = internal standard (cholesterol).

to the view that they need only contain the active principles. In the final analysis, the process used to manufacture the extracts (solvents and extraction methods) is decisive in determining the nature and amount of constituents in the extract (Hänsel, 1990, 1991). In summary, it follows that extract A is not identical with extract B, nor is preparation A identical with preparation B. As with other medicinal plants, there exist ginkgo "total extracts," which are also called "crude extracts or simple extracts" (Fig. 18). They contain most of the constituents in similar ratios as compared with the starting materials. Such extracts are produced mainly using ethanol-water as the extraction medium. The result is a complex mixture of polar to fairly nonpolar natural compounds consisting of active principles, inert plant constituents, and, in some cases, constituents that may cause adverse side effects. In the case of ginkgo, 40 to 60% ethanol is recommended to obtain a high flavonoid yield. A total extract of this type generally contains

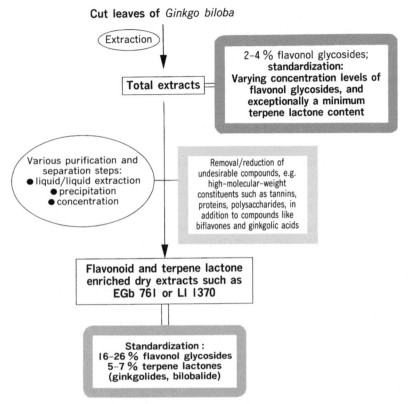

Figure 18. Extraction procedure for and standardization of ginkgo preparations.

2 to 4% ginkgo flavonol glycosides. Commercial products based on total extracts are licensed in a number of European countries for over-the-counter sale.

Furthermore, there are "enriched or special extracts." These products require several steps of purification or separation after extraction and thus possess a higher content of desired constituents, whereas unwanted constitutents are largely eliminated. Ginkgo phytomedicines have been wellknown in Europe, and this is in part due to the development of an enriched or special extract named EGb 761 in the laboratories of Schwabe in Karlsruhe (Germany). This clinically tested ginkgo extract is obtained using a relatively tedious workup and purification procedure, which consists of various steps, such as liquid/liquid extraction, precipitation, and concentration. Therefore, high-molecular-weight constituents, such as tannins, proteins, and polysaccharides, in addition to such compounds as biflavones and ginkgolic acids, are removed or reduced. These substances are undesirable because complex formation can occur with other compounds or they might be allergenic. The desired active principles — namely the flavonoid glycosides and the terpene lactones — are thus enriched. In light of the pharmaceutical and clinical evidence available, use for the indications claimed for the commercial products based on such special extracts usually requires a prescription.

STANDARDIZATION

In the past, all commercially available ginkgo products were adjusted to a given "ginkgo flavone" glycoside content. Products based on the special extracts EGb 761 and LI 1370, such as Tebonin forte (Schwabe), Rökan (Intersan), Tanakan (Ipsen), Ginkobil (Ratiopharm) and Kaveri (Lichtwer Pharma), or products based on extracts manufactured in a similar way, such as Gincosan (ginkgo/ginseng product) (Pharmaton) and Craton (Bioplanta Arzneimittel), are standardized to a ginkgo flavone glycoside content between 16 and 26% w/w. Recently, some individual products of this type also have become standardized on the basis of the presence of 5 to 7% terpene lactones (ginkgolides and bilobalide). Products based on total extracts, such as Valverde Vital (Novartis), Allium Plus (ginkgo/garlic product) (Zeller), and Oxivel (Zeller), are standardized to a flavonoid content of 3.6% w/w and to a minimum terpene lactone content of 0.6%, whereas the French product Arkogelules Ginkgo (Arkopharma) has a minimum flavonoid content of 0.5% w/w.

With reference to the standardization of commercially available products, it should be noted that the declared 16 to 25% w/w ginkgo flavone glycosides and the 5 to 7% w/w terpene lactones, respectively, are related to the extract employed in therapy. For the production of phytomedicines, only an aliquot quantity is used, as, for example, in the case of Tebonin forte solution. Here, 4 g of extract in 100 ml of solution means that the content of the active principles in the phytomedicine is reduced by a factor of 25. However, the view of therapeutic equivalence should be focused more on the daily dosage than on the percentage of active compounds in the extract. For preparations based on EGb 761 extracts, daily dosages that are three times the 40 mg of extract are proposed, which corresponds to 28.6 mg of ginkgo flavonol glycosides and 7.2 mg of terpene lactones. With regard to the use of active constituents for standardization, a reference to flavonol glycosides and terpene lactones not only is desirable, but is absolutely essential.

PHYTOGENERICS

Since the expiration of the patent on extract EGb 761, the question as to whether or not phytomedicine generics—the so-called phytogenerics—exist has been discussed vehemently, because of the lucrative commercial market. Certainly, it can be stated that not all extracts are equal. The manufacturing and production processes leading to an enriched extract, especially in the case of *G biloba*, will include a series of steps in one company that are not likely to be reproducible by another pharmaceutical company. Therefore, the composition of extract constituents and the resulting efficacy may differ. This point is especially important in the case of plant extracts containing more than one active principle (Hänsel, 1990, 1991). The aforementioned facts, however, do not imply that generics are not possible in the area of phytomedicines. If this were the case, phytomedicines would need standards for their registration that well-documented extracts might not satisfy. It is also a fact that differences may exist between generics of synthetically produced substances and the corresponding original medicines. Methods for the comparison of bioavailability exist for generic monosubstances, but are not yet available for phytomedicines. Therefore, a comparable evaluation is much more difficult to perform. In the case of phytomedicines, an evaluation is only possible with comparable proofs of efficacy.

With this point lies the major difficulty in the evaluation of phytomedicines. For ginkgo, no pharmacological or clinical procedures are yet available for leaf extracts. Almost all investigations thus far have involved standardized extracts or their respective preparations, predominantly the previously patented extract EGb 761, and recently also extract LI 1370. Practically all other preparations (an exception is the total extract Zeller; Kade & Miller, 1993), although not manufactured with these extracts, refer to results obtained with EGb 761 and LI 1370. This procedure can by no means be justified. However, it is questionable whether a license for a new ginkgo product with analytically detectable high flavonoid and terpene lactone contents should be refused merely because the manufacturing process did not completely match that of extract EGb 761 or LI 1370, as is currently the practice in Germany. In view of the usual practice in the case of generics, this type of approach would at least represent some novelty. Extension of this practice to phytopharmaceuticals prepared from other plants would have far-reaching consequences for the finished products currently on the market.

CONCLUSIONS

Medicines based on ginkgo leaf extracts have achieved an important role in the treatment of various age-related disorders. Despite extensive studies, ginkgo extract has been at the center of controversy for years, just as are almost all products that are claimed to improve cerebral or peripheral blood flow. Although a positive effect using varied clinical and laboratory parameters has been demonstrated in patients with a cerebro-organic syndrome, further trials in accordance with the modern, strict guidelines for demonstrating the efficacy of nootropics are required.

It would be irresponsible to use ginkgo extracts in advanced peripheral and cerebral circulatory disorders without clarification of the multiple causes by a physician and without medical supervision. For the purpose of stopping or slowing progressive degenerative processes, medication is only one element in a comprehensive therapeutic concept, which must, for example, include memory training in the case of cerebral performance disorders and walking exercise in the case of peripheral blood flow disorders.

Ginkgo products with lower flavonoid or terpene lactone contents that are not claimed to have the same high-level indications as extracts EGb 761 and LI 1370 are licensed for self-medication in a number of European countries, including Switzerland. This raises the question as to whether a special extract with a high content of flavonoids and terpene lactones or a total extract is required for the treatment of primary symptoms of incipient circulatory deficiency. Total extracts are more common in phytotherapy and are the standard with other flavonoid- and proanthocyanidin-containing medicinal plants, as in the case of hawthorn. Dose-finding studies, which could contribute to solving this problem, have not been available. Evidence of therapeutic efficacy is provided by reports that use of total extracts improves both vigilance and mental performance in the elderly. However, carefully performed psychometric studies are still needed to confirm this assertion.

Easily accessible analytical methods for quality control and standardization of both the flavonoids and the terpene lactones are now available to all drug control laboratories. This justifies the requirement of standardized products for the licensing of new ginkgo phytopharmaceuticals. The originally practiced adjustment of flavonol glycosides no longer satisfies the demand for standardization relative to active constituents. Consequently, both the flavonoid and the terpene lactone (ginkgolides and bilobalide) concentrations should be determined in the future. Unstandardized products should no longer be licensed or allowed to remain on the market.

With the expiration of patent protection for EGb 761, the question of generics has arisen. This should not lead to a situation where a new product is not licensed merely because the manufacturing process is not identical to those for extracts EGb 761 and LI 1370. Such an approach would exclude all types of phytogenerics. However, manufacturers of new ginkgo extracts and ginkgo products are expected to develop methods to compare bioavailability. Otherwise, clinical testing of their products should be performed.

REFERENCES

Braquet, P. (Ed.) (1988/1989): *Ginkgolides — Chemistry, Biology, Pharmacology and Clinical* Perspectives. Vols. 1 and 2. Barcelona: Prous.

Briançon-Scheid, F., Guth, A., Anton, R. (1982): High-performance liquid chromatography of biflavones from *Ginkgo biloba* L. *J. Chromatogr.* **245**, 261-267.

Briançon-Scheid, F., Lobstein-Guth, A., Anton, R. (1983): HPLC separation and quantitatlve determination of biflavones in leaves from *Ginkgo biloba*. *Planta Med*. **49**, 204-207.

Camponovo, F.F., Wolfender, J.-L., Maillard, M.P., et al. (1995): Evaporative light scattering and thermospray mass spectrometry: Two alternative mehods for detection and quantitative liquid chromatographic determination of ginkgolides and bilobalode in *Ginkgo biloba* leaf extracts and pytopharmaceuticals. *Phytochem. Anal.* **6**, 141-148.

Carrier, D.-J., Chauret, N., Mancini, M., et al. (1991): Detection of ginkgolide A in *Ginkgo biloba* cell cultures. *Plant Cell Rep.* **10**, 256-259.

Chatterjee, S.S. (1985): Effects of *Ginkgo biloba* extract on cerebral metabolic processes. In: A. Agnoli, J.R. Rapin, V. Scapagnini, W.V. Weitbrecht (Eds.), *Effects of Ginkgo biloba Extract on Organic Cerebral Impairment*. London: John Lebbey Eurotext Ltd.

Chauret, N., Carrier, J., Mancini, M., et al. (1991): Gas chromatographic-mass spectrometric analysis of ginkgolides produced by *Ginkgo biloba* cell culture. *J. Chromatogr.* **588**, 281-287.

DeFeudis, F.V. (1991): *Ginkgo biloba Extract (EGb 761): Pharmacological Activities and Clinical Applications*. Paris: Editions Scientifiques Elsevier.

Flesch, V., Jacques, M., Cosson, L., et al. (1992): Relative importance of growth and light level on terpene content of *Ginkgo biloba*. *Phytochemistry* **31**, 1941- 1945.

Fünfgeld, E.W. (Ed.) (1988): Rökan. *Ginkgo biloba. Recent Results in Pharmacology and Clinic.* Berlin-Heidelberg: Springer-Verlag.

Guth, A., Briançon-Scheid, F., Haag-Berrurier, M., Anton, R. (1981): Analyse qualitative et quantitative des terpènes de *Ginkgo biloba* par HPLC. *Planta Med*. **42**, 129-130.

Hänsel, R. (1990): Analytische Differenzierung verschiedener Ginkgo-Extrakte. Bedeutung des Herstellungsverfahrens für die Extraktzusammensetzung. *Ärzt. Forsch.* **37**, 1-3.

Hänsel, R. (1991): *Ginkgo biloba*: Das Arzneimittelangebot aus pharmazeutischer Sicht. *Apoth. J.* no. 1, 38-42; *Ärzt. Naturheilverfahren* **32**, 295-303.

Hartmann, A., Schulz, V. (Eds.) (1991): *Ginkgo biloba*: Aktuelle Forschungsergebnisse 1990/91.*Münch. Med. Wschr.* **133**, S1-S64.

Hasler, A. (1990): Flavonoide aus *Ginkgo biloba* L. und HPLC-Analytik von Flavonoiden in verschiedenen Arzneipflanzen. Thesis No. 9353, ETH Zurich.

Hasler, A., Meier, B. (1992): Determination of terpenes from *Ginkgo biloba* L. by capillary gas chromatography. *Pharm. Pharmacol. Lett.* **2,** 187-190.

Hasler, A., Meier, B., Sticher, O. (1990a): *Ginkgo biloba*. Botanische, analytische und pharmakologische Aspekte. *Schweiz. Apoth. Ztg*. **28**, 342-347.

Hasler, A., Sticher, O., Meier, B. (1990b): High-performance liquid chromatographic determination of five widespread flavonoid aglycones. *J. Chromatogr.* **508**, 236-240.

Hasler, A., Sticher, O., Meier, B. (1992): Qualitative and quantitative high-performance liquid chromatographic determination of the flavonoids from *Ginkgo biloba. J. Chromatogr.* **605**, 41-48.

Hölzl, J. (1992): Inhaltsstoffe von *Ginkgo biloba. Pharm. Zeit.* **21**, 215-223.

Huh, H., Staba, E.J. (1993): Ontogenetic aspects of ginkgolide production in *Ginkgo biloba. Planta Med.* **59**, 232-239.

Kade, F., Miller, W. (1993): Dose-dependent effects of *Ginkgo biloba* extract on cerebral, mental and physical efficiency — a placebo controlled double blind study. *Br. J. Clin. Res.* **4**, 97-103.

Kleijnen, J., Knipschild, P. (1992a): *Ginkgo biloba. Lancet*, 1136-1139.

Kleijnen, J., Knipschild, P. (1992b): *Ginkgo biloba* for cerebral insufficiency. *Br. J. Clin. Pharmacol.* **34**, 352-358.

Komoda, Y., Nakamura, H., Uchida, M. (1988): HPLC analysis of ginkgolides by using a differential refractometer. *Rep. Inst. Med. Dent. Eng.* **22**, 83-85.

Krieglstein, J. (1994): Neuroprotective properties of *Ginkgo biloba* — constituents. *Zeit. Phytother.* **15**, 92-96.

Lobstein, A., Rietsch-Jako, L., Haag-Berrurier, M., Anton, R. (1991): Seasonal variations of the flavonoid content from *Ginkgo biloba* leaves. *Planta Med.* **57**, 430-433.

Lobstein-Guth, A., Briançon-Scheid, F., Anton, R. (1983): Analysis of terpenes from *Ginkgo biloba* L. by high-performance liquid chromatography. *J. Chromatogr.* **267**, 431-438.

Meier, B., Sticher, O., Bettschart, A. (1985): Weidenrinden-Qualität. Gesamt-salicinbestimmung in Weidenrinden und Weidenpräparaten mit HPLC. *Dtsch. Apoth. Ztg.* **125**, 341-347.

Oberpichler-Schwenk, H., Krieglstein, J. (1992): Pharmakologische Wirkungen von *Ginkgo biloba* — Extrakt und Inhaltsstoffen. *Pharm. Zeit.* **21**, 224-235.

Pietta, P., Mauri, P., Bruno, A., et al. (1991): Identification of flavonoids from *Ginkgo biloba* L., *Anthemis nobilis* L. and *Equisetum arvense* L. by high-performance liquid chromatography with diode-array UV detection. *Planta Med.* **57**, 430-433.

Pietta, P., Mauri, P., Rava, A. (1988): Reversed-phase high-performance liquid chromatographic method for the analysis of biflavones in *Ginkgo biloba* L. extracts. *J. Chromatogr.* **437**, 453-456.

Pietta, P.G., Mauri, P.L., Rava, A. (1990): Analysis of terpenes from *Ginkgo biloba* L. extracts by reversed phase high-performance liquid chromatography. *Chromatographia* **29**, 251-253.

Pietta, P., Mauri, P., Rava, A. (1992): Rapid liquid chromatography of terpenes in *Ginkgo biloba* L. extracts and products. *J. Pharmacol. Biomed. Anal.* **10**, 1077-1079.

Rehwald, A., Meier, B., Sticher, O. (1994): Qualitative and quantitative reversed-phase high-performance liquid chromatography of flavonoids in Crataegus leaves and flowers. *J. Chromatogr. A*, **677**, 25-33.

Schennen, A. (1988): Neue Inhaltsstoffe aus den Blättern von *Ginkgo biloba* L. sowie Präparation ^{14}C-markierter Ginkgo-Flavonoide. Thesis, University of Marburg.

Song, Y. (1986): Chemical composition and utilization of *Ginkgo biloba L. Chem. Ind. Forest Prod.* **6,** (3) 1-4.

Steinke, B., Müller, B., Wagner, H. (1993): Biologische Standardisierungsmethode für Ginkgo-Extrakte. *Planta Med.* **59,** 155-160.

Sticher, O. (1992): *Ginkgo biloba* — Analytik und Zubereitungsformen. *Pharm. Zeit.* **21,** 253-265.

Sticher, O. (1993a): Quality of ginkgo preparations. *Planta Med.* **59,** 2-11.

Sticher, O. (1993b): *Ginkgo biloba* — Ein modernes pflanzliches Arzneimittel. *Vierteljahr. Naturforsch. Gesellschaft Zürich* **138,** 125-168.

Sticher, O., Hasler, A., Meier, B. (1991): *Ginkgo biloba* — eine Standortbestimmung. *Dtsch. Apoth. Ztg.* **131,** 1827-1835.

Tallevi, S.G., Kurz, W.G.W (1991): Detection of ginkgolides by thin-layer chromatography. *J. Nat. Prod.* **54,** 624-625.

Teng, B.P. (1988): Chemistry of ginkgolides. In: P. Braquet (Ed.), *Ginkgolides — Chemistry, Biology, Pharmacology and Clinical Perspectives*, pp. 37-41. Barcelona: Prous.

Van Beek, T.A., Lelyveld, G.P. (1993): Thin-layer chromatography of bilobalide and ginkgolides A, B, C and J on sodium acetate impregnated silica gel. *Phytochem. Anal.* **4,** 109-114.

Van Beek, T.A., Lelyveld, G.P. (1992): Concentration of ginkgolides and bilobalide in *Ginkgo biloba* leaves in relation to the time of year. *Planta Med.* **58,** 413-416.

Van Beek, T.A., Scheeren, H.A., Rantio, T., et al. (1991): Determination of ginkgolides and bilobalide in *Ginkgo biloba* leaves and phytopharmaceuticals. *J. Chromatogr.* **543,** 375-387.

Van Beek, T.A., van Veldhuizen, A., Lelyveld, G.P., et al. (1993): Quantitation of bilobalide and ginkgolides A, B, C and J by means of nuclear magnetic resonance spectroscopy. *Phytochem. Anal.* **4,** 261-268.

Wagner, H., Bladt, S., Hartmann, U., et al. (1989): *Ginkgo biloba.* DC- und HPLC-Analyse von Ginkgo-Extrakten und Ginkgo-Extrakte enthaltenden Phytopräparaten. *Dtsch. Apoth. Ztg.* **129,** 2421-2429.

Wagner, H., Steinke, B. (1991): Biologische Wertbestimmung von Ginkgo-Extrakten. *Münch. Med. Wschr.* **133,** (suppl. 1), S54-S57.

Weber, N. (1986): Platelet activating factor — ein physiologisch aktives Etherlipid. *Pharm. Zeit.* **15,** 107-112.

8

The Herbal Preparations Kangenkaryu and Shen Yun Wan Reduce Brain Oxidative Stress*

Kiminobu Sugaya

Oxidative stress may be a contributing factor to age-related memory dysfunction in some neurodegenerative diseases. Superoxide dismutase (SOD) activity was decreased and lipid peroxides (LPO) were increased in the brain of a senescence-accelerated mouse (SAM) as compared with that of normal senile mice. The goal latency in the water maze was prolonged in SAM, suggesting behavioral impairment. These results indicate that oxidative stress exists in SAM and suggest that it may contribute to the neuronal dysfunction or memory impairment in this mouse model. Kangenkaryu *(KAN) administration (2.25 w/v% in drinking water) partially decreased levels of LPO, but had no effect on SOD activity in SAM.* Shen yun wan *(SYW) administration (12 w/w% in food pellet) increased SOD activity and LPO levels in both SAM and normal senile mice. Combined administration of KAN and SYW elevated the SOD activity and decreased the LPO level to those of the normal senile mice group. In the water maze task, KAN administration decreased the goal latency and SYW enhanced this effect, while SYW alone did not have any effect on the performance of the SAM. Using the $[^{14}C]$-2-deoxyglucose method, KAN administration was shown to increase glucose uptake in the mouse brain. The results indicate that KAN may increase cerebral blood flow, leading to an increase in glucose uptake. When the two herbal drugs were combined, the ability of KAN to reduce*

---

*Some aspects of this review were presented at the 19th CINP meeting, June 27–July 1, 1994, Washington, D.C.

This study was supported by Iskra Industry Co., Ltd. The experiments were performed while the author was at Science University of Tokyo. He wishes to thank Dr. McKinney for his stimulating dialog and support in writing the manuscript.

oxidative stress appeared to be enhanced by SYW, as indicated by a further reduction in LPO levels, perhaps because of the ability of the latter drug to elevate SOD activity and lead to reduced free radicals (superoxide).

INTRODUCTION

The herbal mixture *Kangenkaryu* (KAN) is commonly used to treat many kinds of symptoms related to blood circulation deficiency, based on the theories of Chinese traditional medicine. It appears to decrease blood and plasma viscosity and to dilate blood vessels, leading to an improvement in microcirculation. Therefore, it has been used for the treatment of weakened blood vessels of the brain. KAN is an extract of *Cyperus rhizome, Cnidium rhizome,* peony root, safflower, saussurea root, and salvia root (Jiao, 1990; Takahashi, 1991).

Shen yun wan (SYW) is known as a drug for weak constitutions. It is thought to slow the aging process and to improve the physical constitution when used to treat chronic disease. It is a mixture of *Radix ginseng, Cornu cervi pantotrichum. R angelicae sinensis, R astragali, Fructus lycii, R rehmanniae, Cordyceps, Geeko, Poria, R codonopsis Pilosulae, Rhizoma atractylodis alba, R glycyrrhizae, R dioscoreae, Mel, Oleum sesami* and *Cera flava* (Zhang, 1990).

A well-known animal model of aging that was developed by Takeda et al. (1981), SAM consists of two strains: senescence-accelerated-prone mice (SAM-P) and senescence-accelerated-resistant mice (SAM-R). The latter is the control strain that exhibits normal development and aging characteristics. SAM-P shows an earlier onset and irreversible advancement of senescence, following a normal process of early development. It is characterized by numerous physical signs of aging, including decreased life span and several types of lesions (Takeda et al., 1981; Hosokawa et al., 1986). A systemic amyloidosis occurs in SAM-P (Takeshita et al., 1982). SAM-P/8, a substrain of SAM-P, is known to show a remarkable learning and memory impairment by eight months of age, apparently related to the spontaneous spongi form degeneration of the brain stem (Miyamoto et al., 1986; Yagi et al., 1989). Thus, SAM-P/8 may prove to be a useful model for researching mechanisms related to the memory deficits seen in senile humans.

In this study, the effect of two Chinese traditional medicines, KAN and SYW, alone and in combination (KAN-SYW), on superoxide dismutase (SOD) and brain lipid peroxide (LPO) as oxidative stress markers and memory impairment in SAM-P/8 was examined. SAM-R/1 was studied as the control animal. We also examined the effect of KAN on glucose uptake in the ddY mouse brain, using the $[^{14}C]$ 2-deoxyglucose uptake method.

ANIMAL AND DRUG TREATMENT

Eight to 10 SAM-P/8 and SAM-R/1 mice, 22 to 23 weeks of age at the beginning of the experiments, were used in each group. They were obtained initially from the Department of Pathology, Chest Disease Research Institute, Kyoto University (Takeda et al., 1981). KAN (2.25 w/v%) was dissolved in drinking water and SYW (12 w/w%) was mixed with food pellets for *ad libidum* administration for these experiments. The amount of drug intake, which was calculated by the consumed volume of water or food, was 179.4 ± 8.34 mg per animal per day and 515.6 ± 83.96 mg per animal per day for KAN and SYW respectively.

EFFECTS OF KAN AND SYW

On Memory Performance

The spatial memory testing maze consisted of water ($22 \pm 2°C$; 31 cm deep) in a circular pool made of plastic (80 cm in diameter, 40 cm in height) with a circular escape platform made of transparent acrylic plastic (12 cm in diameter, 30 cm in height). The sessions consisted of four trials, which were performed once a week beginning two weeks after the start of drug administration, and the experimental period was six weeks. At the start of each trial, the mouse was placed in the water and allowed to swim to the platform. Mice not finding the platform within 120 seconds were guided to the platform. The animals were allowed to remain on the platform for 1 minute at the end of each trial. Four different starting positions, equally spaced around the perimeter of the pool, were used, and the platform was located in the center of quadrants defined by these starting positions. The platform and the starting position were fixed in each session and varied in a quasirandom fashion such that the total distance between the points was equal for each session. The behavior of the mice was monitored by a video camera linked to a computer through an image analyzer. The computer (Muromachi Kikai Co., Ltd., Tokyo) calculated the goal latency to escape onto the platform and the swimming speed. Swimming was defined as movement above 1.5 cm per 0.1 second (the sampling time). After the water maze experiment, the mice were sacrificed by decapitation. The brain and liver were dissected out and stored at -80 degress until SOD and LPO were measured.

Untreated SAM-P/8 did not show any progression in goal latency throughout the experiment, while SAM-R/1 showed a gradual decrease in goal latency, indicating learning progress (Fig. 1). The goal latency was significantly decreased in the KAN- treated SAM-P/8 group as compared with the untreated SAM-P/8 mice after three weeks of treatment with the drug. Combined usage

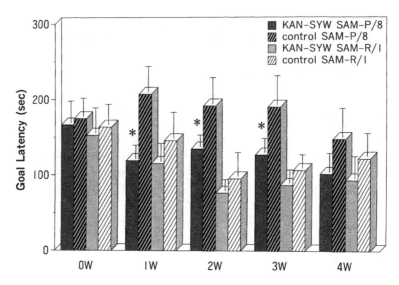

Figure 1. Effect of KAN and SYW administration (four weeks, in combination) on goal latency in the water maze task. SAM-P/8, senescence-accelerated-prone mouse, subline 8; SAM-R/1, senescence-accelerated-resistant mouse, subline 1. The vertical bars represent standard errors of the means ($n = 7$–9). $p < 0.05$, compared with SAM-P/8 control group (Mann-Whitney U test).

with SYW enhanced the effect of KAN (Fig. 1), while SYW by itself did not have any significant effect on goal latency. There were no significant differences in the swimming speed among the four groups. These results suggest that SAM-P/8 exhibits a memory dysfunction by this age, that KAN treatment improves learning in this animal, and that SYW enhances this effect of KAN.

On SOD Activities

The SOD level in the cerebellum was measured by the method of Sichel et al. (1987). The cerebellum was homogenized in nine volumes of 10 mM TRIS-hydrochloric acid (HCl) buffer (pH 7.4) containing 0.32 M sucrose and 1 mM ethylenediamine tetraacidic acid (EDTA). The homogenates were centrifuged and the supernatants were assayed for SOD activity. An aliquot of each sample was retained for determination of protein concentration. The 0.2 ml substrate mixture (1 mM hydroxylamine, 1 mM hypoxanthine) and 0.5 ml purified water were added to Ø.1 ml of sample or 10 mM TRIS-HCl buffer (as a blank). The

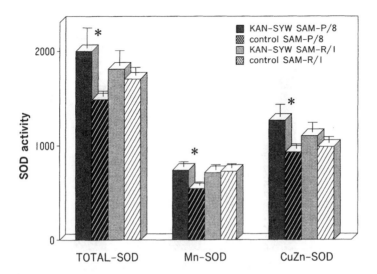

Figure 2. Effect of KAN and SYW administration on SOD activities in the SAMs that were used in the water maze experiment (shown in Fig. 1). For abbreviations, see text and legend to Fig. 1. SOD level was measured in the cerebellum. The vertical bars represent standard errors of the means ($n = 7$–9). $p < 0.05$, compared with SAM-P/8 control group (Student's t-test).

Mn-SOD was assayed in the presence of 2 mM KCN, which selectively inhibits Cu, Zn-SOD. The enzyme solution (6.25 mU/ml XOD (Boehringer-Mannheim; 20 U/ml), 104 mM KH_2PO_4, 78 mM $Na_2B_4O_7$, and 0.5 mM EDTA) was added to the mixture and incubated for 30 minutes at 37°C. After the incubation, 2.0 ml coloring reagent (25% acetic acid containing 0.45 mg/ml sulfanilic acid and 10.4 mg/ml N-1-naphthylethylenediamine) was added and the mixture was allowed to sit at room temperature for 20 minutes. The formation of a colored reaction product was monitored spectrophotometrically at 550 nm (Oyanagui et al., 1984). Under these conditions, one unit of SOD activity is defined as the amount of the enzyme that inhibits the reference rate of reduction of azo dye by 50%.

The levels of both Mn- and Cu,Zn-SOD activity in the cerebellum were significantly decreased in the untreated SAM-P/8 group as compared with the untreated SAM-R/1 group (Fig. 2). In the liver, similar trends were observed, but these did not reach statistical significance (Fig. 3). The KAN treatment slightly increased the level of SOD in SAM-P/8, but not in SAM-R/1, in both the cerebellum and liver. The SYW treatment significantly increased cerebellum and liver levels of SOD activity in both SAM-P/8 and SAM-R/1. Combined usage of

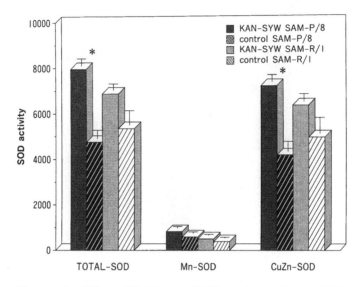

Figure 3. Effect of KAN and SYW administration on SOD activities in the SAMs that were used in the water maze experiment (shown in Fig. 1). For abbreviations, see text and legend to Fig. 1 LPO level was measured in the liver. The vertical bars represent standard errors of the means ($n = 7$-9). $p < 0.05$, compared with SAM-P/8 control group (Student's t-test).

KAN and SYW showed additive effects on SOD activities in aged animals (Figs. 2, 3).

On LPO Levels

The LPO levels in the liver and cerebellum were measured by the method of Mihara and Uchiyama (1983). The liver (about 100 mg) or cerebellum (about 50 mg) was placed in nine volumes of ice-cold 1.15% KCl solution and homogenized with a sonicator. To the sample (0.5 ml) was added 0.3 ml of 1% phosphoric acid solution and 1.0 ml of 0.67% 2-thiobarbituric acid (TBA) solution and the two were mixed. Each aliquot was retained for determination of protein concentration. The test tube was sealed with a glass ball and heated at 95 degrees for 45 minutes. After heating, the tubes were placed on ice and the reaction was stopped by adding 0.4 ml of n-butanol and mixing vigorously. The butanol phase was separated by centrifugation at 3000 rpm for 10 minutes and absorbance in the butanol phase was measured at 535 nm and 520 nm. The difference is a measure of TBA-sensitive LPO levels in the sample. 1,1,3,3-Tetraethoxy propane was used

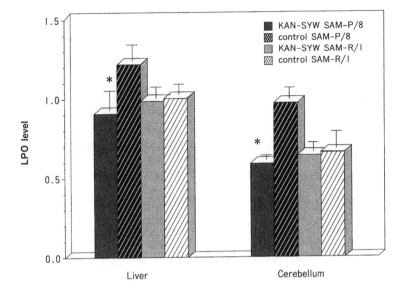

Figure 4. Effect of KAN and SYW administration on LPO levels in the liver and brain of the SAMs that were used in the water maze experiment (shown in Fig. 1). The vertical bars represent standard errors of the means ($n = 7$-9). $p < 0.05$, compared with SAM-P/8 control group (Student's t-test).

as the standard, while saline served as the blank. The corrected TBA value per protein content was regarded as the LPO level for the sample.

The cerebellar LPO level was significantly increased in the untreated SAM-P/8 group as compared with the untreated SAM-R/1 group (Fig. 4). The KAN-SYW treatment had a synergistic effect on the LPO levels in SAM-P/8, reducing them to the level observed in normal senile mice (SAM-R/1) (Fig. 4). These results indicate that KAN-SYW treatment reduces brain oxidative stress, as measured by LPO, in aged animals.

EFFECT OF KAN ON 2-DEOXYGLUCOSE UPTAKE

Four-week-old ddY mice were used for this study. They were housed in cages maintained at 22 ± 2 °C with a 12/12-hour light-dark cycle (lights on at 08.00-20.00 hours). They were divided into three groups saline-treated and two doses of KAN, 100mg and 1000 mg), each containing five mice. KAN was dissolved in saline and administered orally 20 minutes before [^{14}C]2-deoxy- glucose (2DG; 11.8 GBq/mmol, 140 μCi/kg, DuPont NEN) intravenous injection. The mice

(a)   (b)   (c)

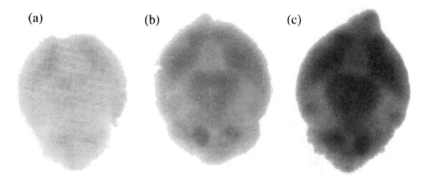

Figure 5. Effect of KAN administration on the glucose uptake in the brain of the ddY mouse. (a) Saline. (b) KAN, 100 mg/animal (by mouth). (c) KAN, 1000 mg/animal (by mouth). The images represent the optical density of film autoradiographs of the brain sections showing [^{14}C]-2-deoxyglucose accumulation. Darker areas represent higher uptake and lighter areas represent lower uptake.

were killed by decapitation. The brains were dissected out and frozen in hexane/dry ice, and 20-μm horizontal sections were obtained. The sections were placed on plastic tapes and juxtaposed to X-ray film (SR-2, Kodak) with an autoradiographic [^{14}C] microscale (Amersham) for three weeks at room temperature. Autoradiographic films exposed to brain sections were scanned with an Epson GT-800 scanner and digitized images were printed using a Quadra 840AV (Macintosh).

KAN dose-dependently increased glucose uptake in the brains of ddY mice (Fig. 5). This may result from an increase in cerebral blood flow, but a direct stimulatory action of KAN on neurons is also possible.

CONCLUSION

Orally administered KAN dose-dependently increased glucose uptake in the ddY mouse brain. This may indicate an increase in cerebral blood flow, since KAN is known to decrease blood viscosity (Igarashi et al., 1986). In the SAM-P/8, the administration of KAN-SYW led to a decrease in goal latency in the water maze task, indicating improved learning, and the drug altered levels of SOD activity and LPO content to levels similar to those of the normal senile mouse. We speculate that KAN may increase cerebral blood flow, while SYW may directly stimulate cells to increase SOD activity. Increased blood flow and SOD activity may help decrease oxidative stress in aging, thus preserving brain function and improving behavior. These results indicate that KAN and SYW contain one or more active principles capable of altering brain function in a way relevant to the pharmacotherapy of senile dementia.

REFERENCES

Hosokawa, M., Kasai, R., Higuchi, K. (1986) : Grading score system: A method for evaluation of the degree of senescence in senescence accelerated mouse (SAM). *Mech. Aging Dev.* **26**, 91-102.

Igarashi, M., Kanno, H., Tanaka, K., et al. (1986): Preventive function of substances in the pyrazine class against blood platelet aggregation. *J. Med. Soc. Toho University* **33**, 261-264 (Abstract. in English)

Jiao, D.H. (1990): Clinical trial test of Kanjin II in Gou Shi Kui Chinese Medical Center of Aging. *Chin. Trad. Patent Med.* **12**, 23.

Mihara, M., and Uchiyama, M. (1983): Properties of thiobarbituric acid-reactive materials obtained from lipid peroxide and tissue homogenate. *Chem. Pharmaceut. Bull.* **31**, 605-611.

Miyamoto, M., Kiyota, Y., Yamazaki, N. (1986): Age-related changes in learning and memory in the senescence-accelerated mouse (SAM). *Physiol. Behav.* **38**, 399-406.

Oyanagui, Y. (1984): Reevaluation of assay method and establishment of kit for superoxide dismutase activity. *Ana,. Biochem.* **142**, 290-296.

Sichel, G., Corsaro, C., Scalia, M. Geremia, E. (1987): Relationship between melanin content and superoxide dismutase (SOD) activity in the liver of various species of animals. *Cell Biochem. Function* **5**, 123-128.

Takahashi, H. (1991): Clinical trial of prescription of *Kaketsukeo. Clin. J. Chinese Med.* **12**, 145-151.

Takeda, T., Hosokawa, M., Takeshita, S. (1981): A new murine model of accelerated senescence. *Mech. Aging Dev.* **17**, 183-194.

Takeshita, S., Hosokawa, M., Irino, M. (1982): Spontaneous age-associated amyloidosis in senescence-accelerated mouse (SAM). *Mech. Ageing Dev.* **20**, 13-23.

Yagi, H., Irino. M., Matsushima, T., Takeda, T. (1989): Spontaneous spongy degeneration of the brain stem in SAM-P/8 mice, a newly developed memory-deficient strain. *J. Neuropathol. Exp. Neurol.* **48**, 577-590.

Zhang, E. (1990): *English-Chinese Highly Efficacious Chinese Patent Medicines.* Shanghai: Publishing House of Shanghai College of Traditional Chinese Medicine.

9

Effect of Herbal Medicine on Learning Disturbances in Senescence-Accelerated Mice

Masao Kishikawa

Japanese herbal medicines, or Kampo, *basically reflect the traditions of Chinese medicine, but in the course of their use over hundreds of years, they have developed into a product that is uniquely Japanese. It is necessary now to take their use one step further on the basis of this long experience and to conduct a more scientific investigation concerning their effects.*

The herbal medicine Toki-shakuyaku-san *(TSS), is an extract of six types of herbs (Table 1) that has been used traditionally for a wide range of gynecologic diseases, such as ovarian insufficiency and endometriosis. TSS was also recently reported to have a useful pharmacologic effect on neural transmitters in the brain (Koyama, 1989).*

The investigation of the effects of TSS on the behavior, learning ability, and histologic changes in animals may be important for basic studies concerning the prevention and treatment of senile dementia in humans.

MATERIALS AND METHODS

Experimental Animals

The male senescence-accelerated mouse (SAM), which was originally developed by Dr. T. Takeda (Institute for Thoracic Diseases, Kyoto University, Japan), displays a number of symptoms similar to those observed in human aging

The author expresses his appreciation to Ms. Sakae and Dr. Kondo, Scientific Data Center, and Dr. Sato and Mr. Sasano, Laboratory Animal Center, Nagasaki University, for their invaluable cooperation. The TSS, *Toki-Shakuyaku-San* (Tsumura TJ-23), was provided by Tsumura & Co., Tokyo, Japan. This study was supported, in part, by a grant from Tsumura & Co.

TABLE 1

Composition of TSS*

Ingredients (herbs)	Components
Angelicae radix (3 g)	Ligustiide, n-butylidenphthalide, sedanoic acid, safrol, palmitic acid, linolic acid, bergaptene, scopoletin, falcarinol, falcarindiol, vitamin B_{12}, nicotic acid
Paeoniae radix (4 g)	Paeoniflorin, oxypaeoniflorin, benzoyl paeoniflorin, albiflorin, paeonol
Cnidii rhizoma (3 g)	Ligustilide, cnidilide, neocnidilide, butylphthalide, butylidenephthalide
Atractylodis Lanceae rhizoma (4 g)	Hinesol, β-eudesmol, elemol, atractylodin
Alismatis rhizoma (4 g)	Alisol A, B, C, alisol A, B, C monoacetate, D-glucose, D-fructose, sucrose, β-sitosterol, lecithin, choline
Hoelen (4 g)	Pachyman, eburicoic acid, pachymic acid, dehydroeburicoic acid, ergosterol, 3β-o-acetyltumulosic acid, 3β-o-acetyldehydrotumulosic acid

* This recipe is used to produce 4.0 g of TSS extract, which is the daily dose for humans (80 mg/kg/day).

(Takeda et al., 1981). The present study employed the SAM substrain SAMP1TA/Ngs (Kishikawa et al., 1994) raised in more than 20 successive generations under conventional clean conditions in the Laboratory Animal Center at Nagasaki University. The 43 mice included a group of 21 mice receiving TSS (treated group) and 22 untreated mice (control group).

Method of Administration

Pellet feed (CE-2, Nihon CLEA, Tokyo) containing 0.044% TSS (Tsumura & Co., Tokyo; TJ-23), or a total dose of 80 mg/kg/day, was given to the treated group *ad libitum* from the age of six weeks for 10 weeks and 24 weeks.

Learning Ability and Behavior

The assessment of learning ability and behavior was conducted just before sacrifice at the age of four or seven months. Learning ability was assessed by the Morris, water maze test (Morris, 1981) and the step-down passive avoidance task (Nishimura et al., 1990), while spontaneous motor activity was measured using a tilting-type ambulometer (Kishikawa et al.,1993). The tests were carried out on each mouse in the above order, but with an interval of at least one day between tests.

The Morris water maze test was administered twice a day for three days at the same time in the afternoon. Each time, the mouse was dropped into the water at four separate points (at 90-degree intervals) around the edge of a circular tub. The mice were then allowed to swim and to escape onto a hidden platform in the tub. The time that elapsed from immersion to arrival at the platform was measured. The limit was 120 seconds. The pillar holding the platform was fixed at the center of one quadrant of the circular tub. The top of the platform was 1 cm below the surface of the water, which was mixed with milk for camouflage.

The single-trial step-down passive avoidance task consisted of two phases. In the first phase, or training trial, a 0.4 mA electric shock of 2 seconds, duration was applied to the feet of each mouse as it stepped down onto the grid floor. The mice were immediately returned to their cages after only one training trial. In the second phase of the task, or test trial, conducted 24 hours later, each mouse was again placed on the platform, and the latent period from the placing of the mouse on the platform to the point when the mouse stepped down onto the grid floor was measured. In this test trial, the maximum latent period was set at 180 seconds for standard achievement.

The seven-month-old TSS-treated group that underwent treatment for 24 weeks was subjected not only to a single trial, but also to electric shock from the second day on in order to determine on what day the mice reached the standard achievement of 180 seconds.

Spontaneous motor activity was measured using a tilting-type ambulometer. Each mouse was placed in a separate experimental bucket, and the number of vibrations was recorded every 10 minutes for a period of 150 minutes.

Morphologic examination

Soon after the measurement of behavior, the mice were sacrificed under nembutal anaesthesia. After fixation, 8 μm light microscope specimens were made from the sections of the hippocampus and other regions. After hemotoxylin and eosin, periodic acid-Schiff (PAS) and myelin staining, the sections were examined histologically. A morphometric study was carried out using an image

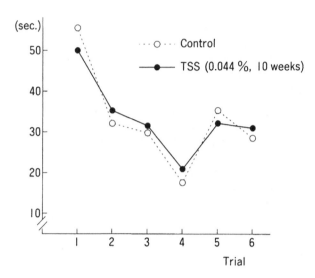

Figure 1. Water maze task response. In the 10-week feeding experiment, the TSS-treated group and the control group scored an average of 30.9 and 28.7 seconds, respectively, in the last trial on the third day.

analysis processor (nexusQube; Nexus Inc., Japan). An electron microscopic study was also conducted.

Statistical Analysis

In the statistical study, we used a method of normal survival time analysis called the log rank test, as well as Wilcoxon's rank sum test.

RESULTS

Learning Ability

Morris Water Maze Task: In the 10-week feeding groups, the TSS-treated group and the control group scored an average of 50 and 52 seconds, respectively, on the first trial on the first day. On the last trial on the third day, they scored 31 and 29 seconds respectively (Fig.1). In the groups fed TSS for 24 weeks, the TSS-treated group and the control group scored an average of 46.5 and 61.0 seconds, respectively, on the first trial on the first day. On the last trial on the third day, they scored 16.9 and 23.0 seconds respectively.

There was no significant statistical difference between the two groups, even at different ages.

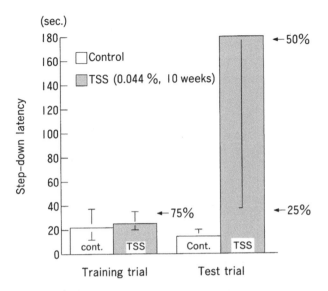

Figure 2. Single-trial step–down latency.

Passive Avoidance Task: On the training trial on the first day, the latent period was short in both groups at each age, and there was no significant statistical difference between the treated group and the control group. On the test trial, however, the latent period was 15 seconds for the control group but 179 seconds for the group treated with TSS for 10 weeks (Fig. 2). The test trial revealed a tremendous statistical difference between the two groups (Fig. 3).

The seven-month-old mice that underwent treatment for 24 weeks were subjected not only to a single trial, but from the second day on also to electric shock when they stepped down. The day on which the mice reached the standard achievement of 180 seconds was determined. There was no statistically significant difference in the latent period for the first test trial on the second day between the treated group and the control group.

Although the control groups required seven days to acquire learning, the treated groups seemed to require only three to four days for the acquisition of learning ability (Fig. 4).

Spontaneous Motility: Throughout the 150-minute experiment, the amount of activity every 10 minutes seemed to be almost the same, and there was no significant statistical difference between the treated group and the control group at any point (Fig. 5).

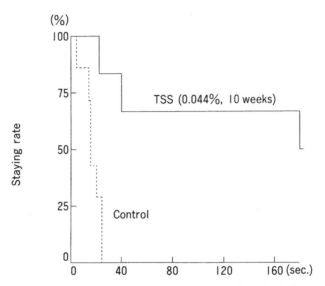

Figure 3. Step-down latency by the method of survival time analysis in the test trial. There was a significant difference between the 0.044% TSS-treated group and the control group ($p < 0.01$).

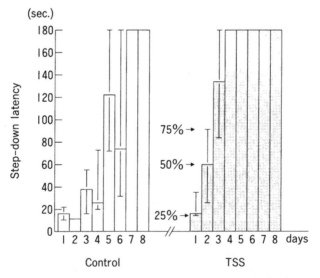

Figure 4. Step-down task response in the 24-week-feeding experiment. Although the control groups required seven days for acquisition, the treated groups seemed to require only three to four days. ☐: control group, ▨: 0.044% TSS (10-week) treated group.

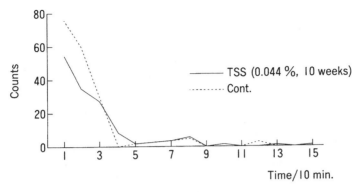

Figure 5. Spontaneous motility. There was no significant statistical difference between the treated group and the control group.

Morphology

There was no notable difference in the weight of the brain or other features between the treated group and the control group.

On the light microscopic level, there was no particular histopathologic difference between the two groups in the 10-week-feeding experiment. In the 24-week-feeding experiment, however, PAS-positive granular structures (PPGSs) as minute as 5 μm were frequently scattered in the hippocampus of the control group. These PPGSs were also present, although in much smaller amounts, in the hippocampus of the treated group. Small to minute vacuolar changes were observed from the midbrain to the medulla oblongata, with particular prominence in the pontine reticular formation. On the electron microscopic level, these tiny vacuoles might correspond to the degenerative alterations of the myelin sheath and/or postsynaptic portions. The mean number of vacuoles in the pontine reticular formation was 43.7 ± 30.7 in the treated group but 81.3 ± 33.5 in the control group (Table 2). Although not actually significant, the *p*-value of 0.07 between the two groups reflects a difference very close to statistical significance.

DISCUSSION

An effective remedy for senile dementia has not been established despite remarkable developments in the field of neuroscience. One of the reasons for this delay is the fact that the actual pathogenesis of senile dementia remains obscure, but another important obstacle to the elucidation and treatment of senile dementia is said to be the lack of a useful animal model (Kishikawa et al., 1993; Games et

TABLE 2

Morphometrical data of vacuoles in the pontine
reticular formation.*

Area (μm^2)	Control	TSS
- 10	16.2± 8.6	8.0± 6.6
10- 20	13.7± 6.7	6.7± 4.4
20- 30	5.7± 5.1	3.3± 3.4
30- 40	6.8± 4.3	3.8± 4.2
40- 50	4.7± 2.3	1.8± 2.0
50- 60	2.3± 1.6	2.7± 1.8
60- 70	2.5± 1.5	1.0± 1.3
70- 80	4.0± 3.0	1.0± 1.3
80- 90	3.8± 2.6	1.5± 1.4
90-100	3.0± 1.1	2.2± 2.9
100-	18.7± 7.0	11.7±11.2
Total number	81.3±33.5	43.7±30.7

* The changes seem to be particularly prominent in the control group.

al., 1995). SAM, a mouse that exhibits accelerated senescence, was developed by
Takeda more than a decade ago (Takeda et al., 1981). Although spontaneously
occurring learning and memory disturbances are well known in SAMP8 and
SAMP10 (Miyamoto et al., 1986; Shimada et al., 1992), it is also reported that
the substrain SAMP1TA/Ngs exhibits a learning disturbance without amyloid
deposition (Kishikawa et al., 1994). The learning disturbance in SAMP8 is
characterized by an onset at two months of age and subsequent progression with
age. In contrast, SAMP1TA/Ngs displays a high level of learning behavior at
around five months of age and subsequently suffers a loss of learning ability due
to accelerated senescence. The increase up to the age of five months and subsequent decrease in dendritic spines in the rapid Golgi study may be evidence of
the behavioral pattern of learning in SAMP1TA/Ngs, reflecting the process by
which learning ability, once acquired, is impaired by accelerated senescence
(Kawaguchi et al., 1994). This pattern resembles the process of brain dysfunction
appearing in human beings as a result of senescence. This is the reason why we
selected the substrain SAMP1TA/Ngs from among the strains of SAM for this
study.

It is extremely interesting that, in the study of passive avoidance ability, a
prominent acquisition disability appeared in the nontreated control group.
Considering the fact that there was no difference in spontaneous motor activity
between the treated and control groups, it is unlikely that a difference in

spontaneous activity on the platform affected the latent period. In other words, it is unlikely that a dulling of the activity of SAM due to TSS prolonged the latent period in the test trial and/or latent step-down period.

The learning-disturbance-like behavior observed in SAMP1TA/Ngs can be categorized into two patterns: (1) disturbance in the acquisition of learning ability at around three months of age due to immaturity of the neuronal network, especially dendritic spines (Kawaguchi et al., 1994); and (2) learning disturbance at seven months of age as a result of accelerated senescence. The favorable results on the one-trial passive avoidance task in the group treated for 10 weeks suggest that the ongoing development of dendritic spines is promoted by TSS at around three months of age.

The extent of morphologic changes such as PPGSs and vacuolar changes of the reticular formation in the brain stem was relatively indistinct in the treated group. It is reported that PPGSs observed at the light microscopic level corresponded to abnormal synaptic terminals (Irino et al., 1994). We also have information suggesting that the PPGSs corresponds to the postsynaptic terminal of neuronal dendrites (unpublished data). Although TSS has been used traditionally for a wide range of gynecologic diseases, it was recently reported to have a useful pharmacologic effect on neural transmitters in the brain (Koyama, 1989). It is also known that the nuclei in the reticular formation of the brain stem have long and ascending projections to the limbic system and cerebral cortex, with a significant relation to learning and memory (Takeda et al., 1991; Kornblith & Olds, 1973; Gabriel et al., 1986). Septal and commissural fibers terminate at the dendrites of hippocampal pyramidal neurons. Septal nuclei also receive information from the brain stem, particularly its reticular formation (Vertes, 1985). These facts strongly suggest that vacuolar changes, PPGSs, and learning ability are interrelated. TSS seems to play an important role in preventing the impairment of the synaptic device and in repairing the synaptic transmitting system.

It is important to evaluate the morphometry of the dendritic spines in the hippocampal pyramidal neurons in this TSS-feeding study, because the SAMP1TA/Ngs used in our experiments demonstrate an intimate correlation between the results of the step-down passive avoidance task and the number of dendritic spines in the hippocampal CA1 pyramidal neurons (Kawaguchi et al., 1994).

REFERENCES

Gabriel, M., Gregg. B., Clancy, A., et al. (1986): Brain stem reticular formation neuronal correlates of stimulus significance and behavior during discriminative avoidance conditioning in rabbits. *Behav. Neurosci.* **100**(2), 171-184.

Games, D., Adams, D., Alessandeini, R., et al. (1995): Alzheimer-type neuropathology in transgenic mice overexpressing V717F β-amyloid precursor protein. *Nature* **373** (6514), 523-527.

Irino, M., Akiguchi. I., Takeda, T. (1994): Ultrastructural study of PAS-positive granular structures (PGS) in brains of SAMP8. In: T. Takeda (Ed.), *The SAM Model of Senescence*, 371-374. Amsterdam: Elsevier Science.

Kawaguchi, S., Kishikawa, M., Ikematsu, K., et al. (1994): Age-related changes in hippocampal pyramidal cells (CA1) among SAMP1TA/Ngs-A quantitative rapid Golgi study of basal dendrites and dendritic spines. In : T. Takeda (Ed.), *The SAM Model of Senescence*, 331-333. Amsterdam: Elsevier Science.

Kishikawa, M., Nishimura, M., Sakae, M., Iseki, M. (1993): The learning ability and motility of senescence accelerated mice (SAM-P/1) treated with *Toki-shakuyaku-san*. *Phytother. Res.* **7**, S63-S66.

Kishikawa, M., Sakae, M., Iseki, M., et al. (1994): Ecology and learning ability of SAMP1TA/Ngs raised at Nagasaki. In: T. Takeda (Ed.), *The SAM Model of Senescence*, 381-384. Amsterdam: Elsevier Science.

Kornblith, C., Olds, J. (1973): Unit activity in brain stem reticular formation of the rat during learning. *J. Neurophysiol.* **36**(3), 489-501.

Koyama, T. (1989): Effects of *Toki-shakuyaku-san* on neurotransmitter in the brain. *Gendai Iryogaku* **14**, 89-95 (in Japanese).

Miyamoto, M., Kiyota, Y., Yamazaki, N., et al. (1986): Age-related changes in learning and memory in the senescence-accelerated mouse (SAM). *Physiol. Behav.* **38**, 399-406.

Morris, R.G.M. (1981): Spatial localization does not require the presence of local cues. *Learn. Motiv.* **12**, 239-260.

Nishimura, M., Shiigi, Y., Kaneto, H. (1990): State dependent and/or direct memory retrieval by morphine in mice. *Psychopharmacology* **100**, 27-30.

Shimada, A., Ohta, A., Akiguchi, I., Takeda, T. (1992): Inbred SAM-P/10 as a mouse model of spontaneous, inherited brain atrophy. *J. Neuropathol. Exp. Neurol*. **51**: 440-450.

Takeda, T., Hosokawa, M., Takeshita, S. et al. (1981): A new murine model of accelerated senescence. *Mech. Ageing. Dev.* **17**, 183-194.

Takeda, T., Hosokawa, M., Higuchi, K. (1991): Senescence-accelerated mouse (SAM) : A novel murine model of accelerated senescence. *J. Am. Geriatr. Soc.* **39**(9), 911-919.

Vertes, R.P. (1985): Brainstem-septohippocampal circuits controlling the hippocampal EEG. In: G. Buzsaki, C.H. Vanderwolf (Eds.), *Electrical Activity of the Archicortex*, 33-45. Budapest: Akademiai Kiado.

Subject Index

T - #0590 - 101024 - C0 - 212/152/8 - PB - 9780876308042 - Gloss Lamination